The Ultimate Alkaline Diet Guide for Beginners

Amazing and Affordable Recipes to Make Incredible Salads and Smoothies

Bella Francis

Table of contents

Kale Pesto's Pasta

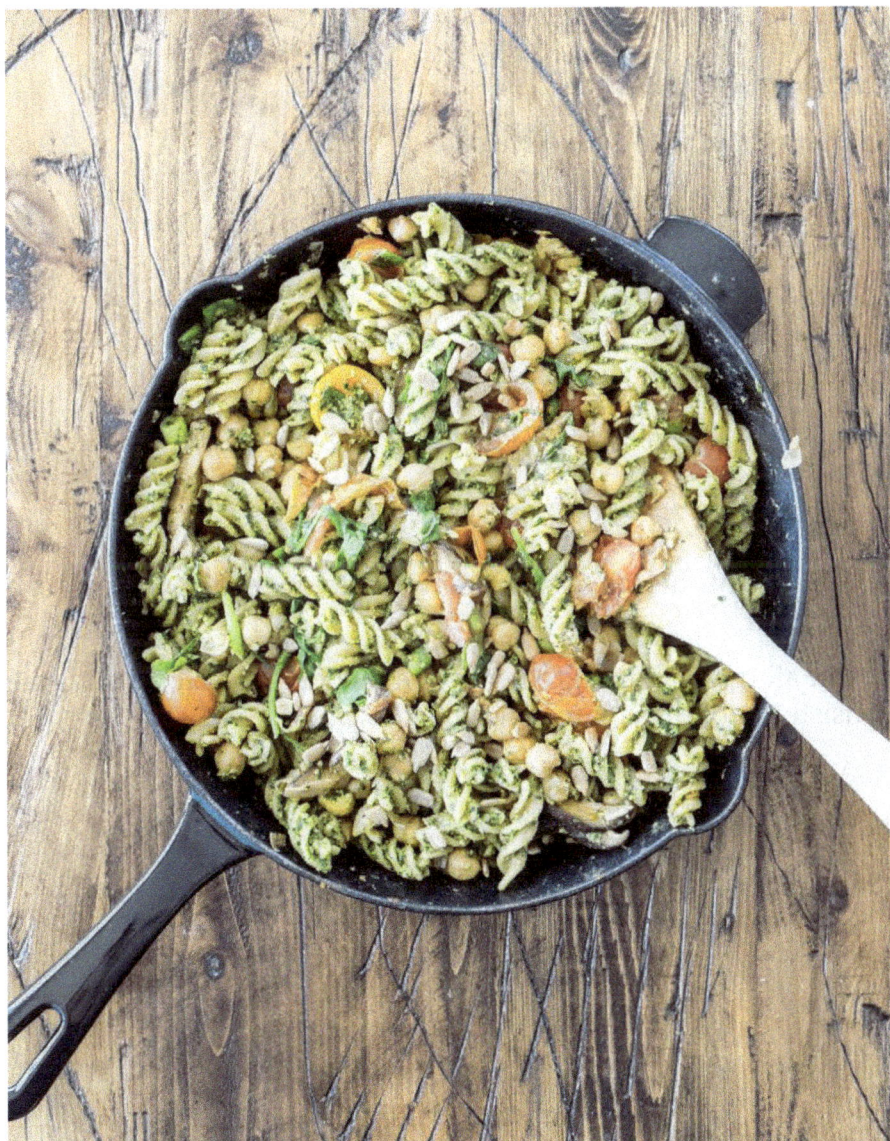

Preparation Time: 10 minutes

Cooking Time: 0 minutes

Servings: 1-2

Ingredients :

- 1 bunch of kale
- 2 cups of fresh basil
- 1/4 cup of extra virgin olive oil
- 1/2 cup of walnuts
- 2 limes, freshly squeezed
- Sea salt and chili pepper
- 1 zucchini, noodle (spiralizer)
- Optional: garnish with chopped asparagus, spinach leaves, and tomato.

Directions:

1. The night before, soak the walnuts in order to improve absorption.

2. Put all the recipe Ingredients in a blender and blend until the consistency of the cream is reached.

3. Add the zucchini noodles and enjoy.

Nutrition:

Calories: 55

Carbohydrates: 9 g

Fat: 1.2g

Cranberry And Brussels Sprouts With Dressing

Preparation Time: 10 minutes

Cooking Time: 0 minute

Servings: 4

Ingredients :

Ingredients for the dressing

- ⅓ cup extra-virgin olive oil

- 2 tbsp. apple cider vinegar

- 1 tbsp. pure maple syrup

- Juice of 1 orange

- ½ tbsp. dried rosemary

- 1 tbsp. scallion, whites only

- Pinch sea salt

For the salad

- 1 bunch scallions, greens only, finely chopped

- 1 cup Brussels sprouts, stemmed, halved, and thinly sliced

- ½ cup fresh cranberries

- 4 cups fresh baby spinach

Directions:

1. To make the dressing: In a bowl, whisk the dressing Ingredients.

2. To make the salad: Add the scallions, Brussels sprouts, cranberries, and spinach to the bowl with the dressing.

3. Combine and serve.

Nutrition:

Calories: 267

Fat: 18g

Carbohydrates: 26g

Protein: 2g

Sebi's Vegetable Salad

Preparation Time: 10 minutes

Cooking Time: 0 minutes

Servings: 1-2

Ingredients :

• 4 cups each of raw spinach and romaine lettuce

• 2 cups each of cherry tomatoes, sliced cucumber, chopped baby carrots and chopped red, orange and yellow bell pepper

• 1 cup each of chopped broccoli, sliced yellow squash, zucchini and cauliflower.

Directions:

1. Wash all these vegetables.

2. Mix in a large mixing bowl and top off with a non-fat or low-fat dressing of your choice.

Nutrition:

Calories: 48

Carbohydrates: 11g

Protein: 3g

Sebi's Alkaline Spring Salad

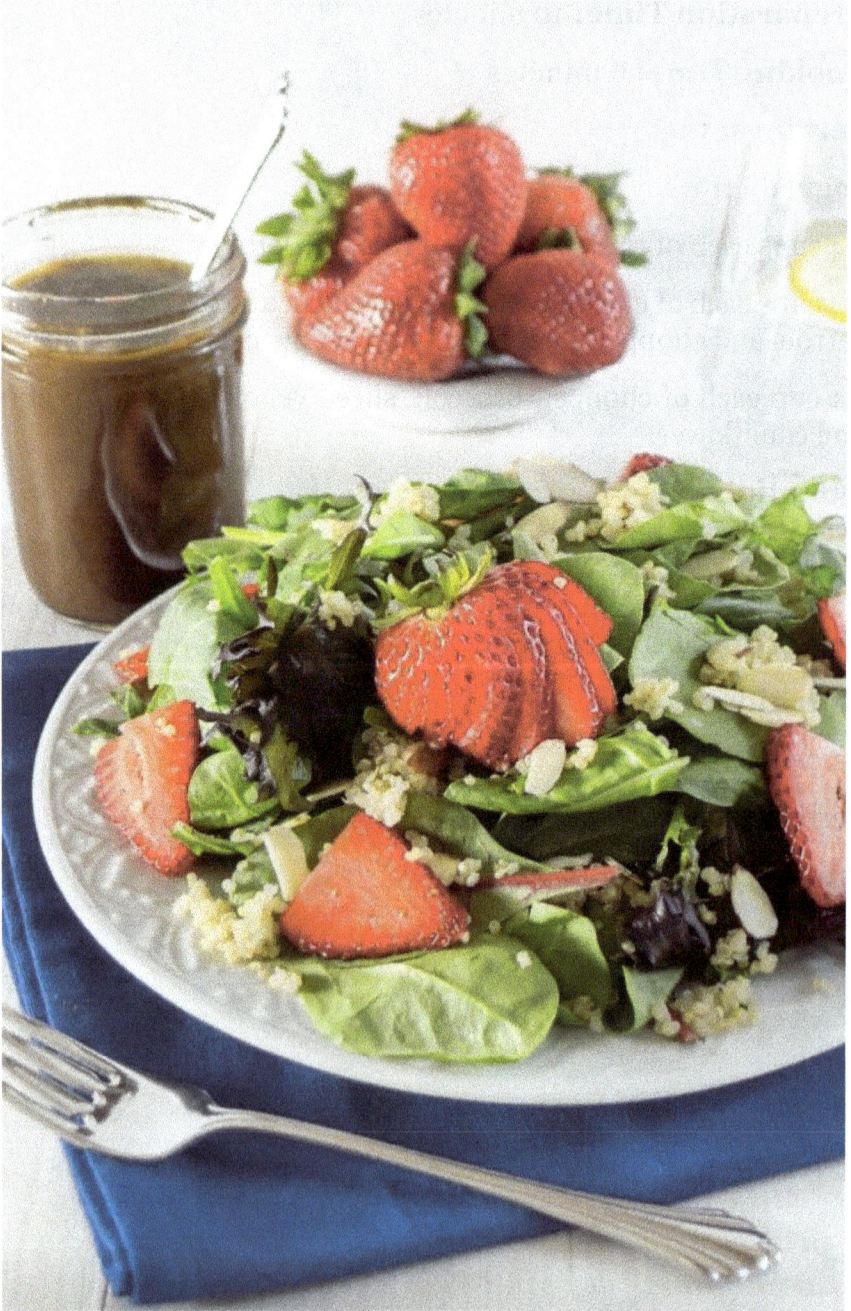

Preparation Time: 10 minutes

Cooking Time: 0 minutes

Servings: 1-2

Eating seasonal fruits and vegetables is a fabulous way of taking care of yourself and the environment at the same time. This alkaline-electric salad is delicious and nutritious.

Ingredients :

• 4 cups seasonal approved greens of your choice

• 1 cup cherry tomatoes

• 1/4 cup walnuts

• 1/4 cup approved herbs of your choice

• For the dressing:

• 3-4 key limes

• 1 tbsp. of homemade raw sesame

• Sea salt and cayenne pepper

Directions:

1. First, get the juice of the key limes. In a small bowl, whisk together the key lime juice with the homemade raw sesame "tahini" butter. Add sea salt and cayenne pepper, to taste.

2. Cut the cherry tomatoes in half.

3. In a large bowl, combine the greens, cherry tomatoes , and herbs. Pour the dressing on top and "massage" with your hands.

4. Let the greens soak up the dressing. Add more sea salt, cayenne pepper, and herbs on top if you wish. Enjoy!

Nutrition:

Calories: 77

Carbohydrates: 11g

Thai Quinoa Salad

Preparation Time: 10 minutes

Cooking Time: 0 minutes

Servings: 1-2

Ingredients :

Ingredients used for dressing:

- 1 tbsp. Sesame seed
- 1 tsp. Chopped garlic
- 1 tsp. Lemon, fresh juice
- 3 tsp. Apple Cider Vinegar
- 2 tsp. Tamari, gluten-free.
- 1/4 cup of tahini (sesame butter)
- 1 pitted date
- 1/2 tsp. Salt
- 1/2 tsp. toasted Sesame oil

Salad Ingredients:

- 1 cup of quinoa, steamed
- 1 big handful of arugula
- 1 tomato cut in pieces
- 1/4 of the red onion, diced

Directions:

1. Add the following to a small blender: 1/4 cup + 2 tbsp.

2. Filtered water, the rest of the Ingredients. Blend, man. Steam 1 cup of quinoa in a steamer or a rice pan, then set aside.

3. Combine the quinoa, the arugula, the tomatoes sliced, the red onion diced on a serving plate or bowl, add the Thai dressing

4. and serve with a spoon.

Nutrition:

Calories: 100

Carbohydrates: 12 g

Green Goddess Bowl And Avocado Cumin Dressing

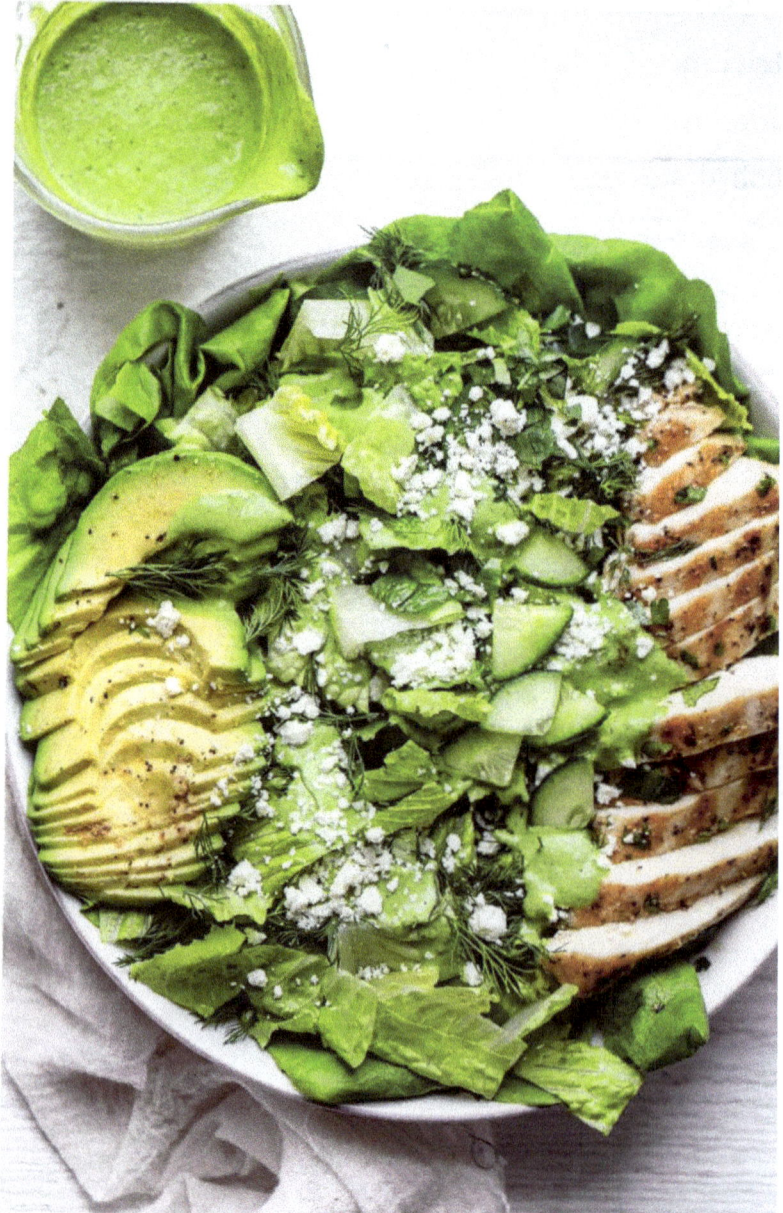

Preparation Time: 10 minutes

Cooking Time: 0 minutes

Servings: 1-2

Ingredients :

Ingredients for the dressing of avocado cumin:

- 1 Avocado
- 1 tbsp. Cumin Powder
- 2 limes, freshly squeezed
- 1 cup of filtered water
- 1/4 seconds. sea salt
- 1 tbsp. Olive extra virgin olive oil
- Cayenne pepper dash
- Optional: 1/4 tsp. Smoked pepper

Tahini Lemon Dressing Ingredients

- 1/4 cup of tahini (sesame butter)
- 1/2 cup of filtered water (more if you want thinner, less thick)
- 1/2 lemon, freshly squeezed
- 1 clove of minced garlic
- 3/4 tsp. Sea salt (Celtic Gray, Himalayan, Redmond Real Salt)
- 1 tbsp. Olive extra virgin olive oil
- black pepper taste

Salad Ingredients:

- 3 cups of kale, chopped
- 1/2 cup of broccoli flowers, chopped
- 1/2 zucchini (make spiral noodles)

- 1/2 cup of kelp noodles, soaked and drained

- 1/3 cup of cherry tomatoes, halved.

- 2 tsp. hemp seeds

Directions:

1. Gently steam the kale and the broccoli (flash the steam for 4 minutes), set aside.

2. Mix the zucchini noodles and kelp noodles and toss with a generous portion of the smoked avocado cumin dressing. Add the cherry tomatoes and stir again.

3. Place the steamed kale and broccoli and drizzle with the lemon tahini dressing. Top the kale and the broccoli with the noodles and tomatoes and sprinkle the whole dish with the hemp seeds.

Nutrition:

Calories: 89

Carbohydrates: 11g

Fat: 1.2g

Protein: 4g

Sweet And Savory Salad

Preparation Time: 10 minutes

Cooking Time: 0 minutes

Servings: 1-2

Ingredients :

- 1 big head of butter lettuce
- 1/2 of cucumber, sliced
- 1 pomegranate, seed or 1/3 cup of seed
- 1 avocado, 1 cubed
- 1/4 cup of shelled pistachio, chopped

Ingredients for dressing:

- 1/4 cup of apple cider vinegar
- 1/2 cup of olive oil
- 1 clove of garlic, minced

Directions:

1. Put the butter lettuce in a salad bowl.

2. Add the remaining Ingredients and toss with the salad dressing.

Nutrition:

Calories: 68

Carbohydrates: 8g

Fat: 1.2g

Protein: 2g

Beet Salad With Basil Dressing

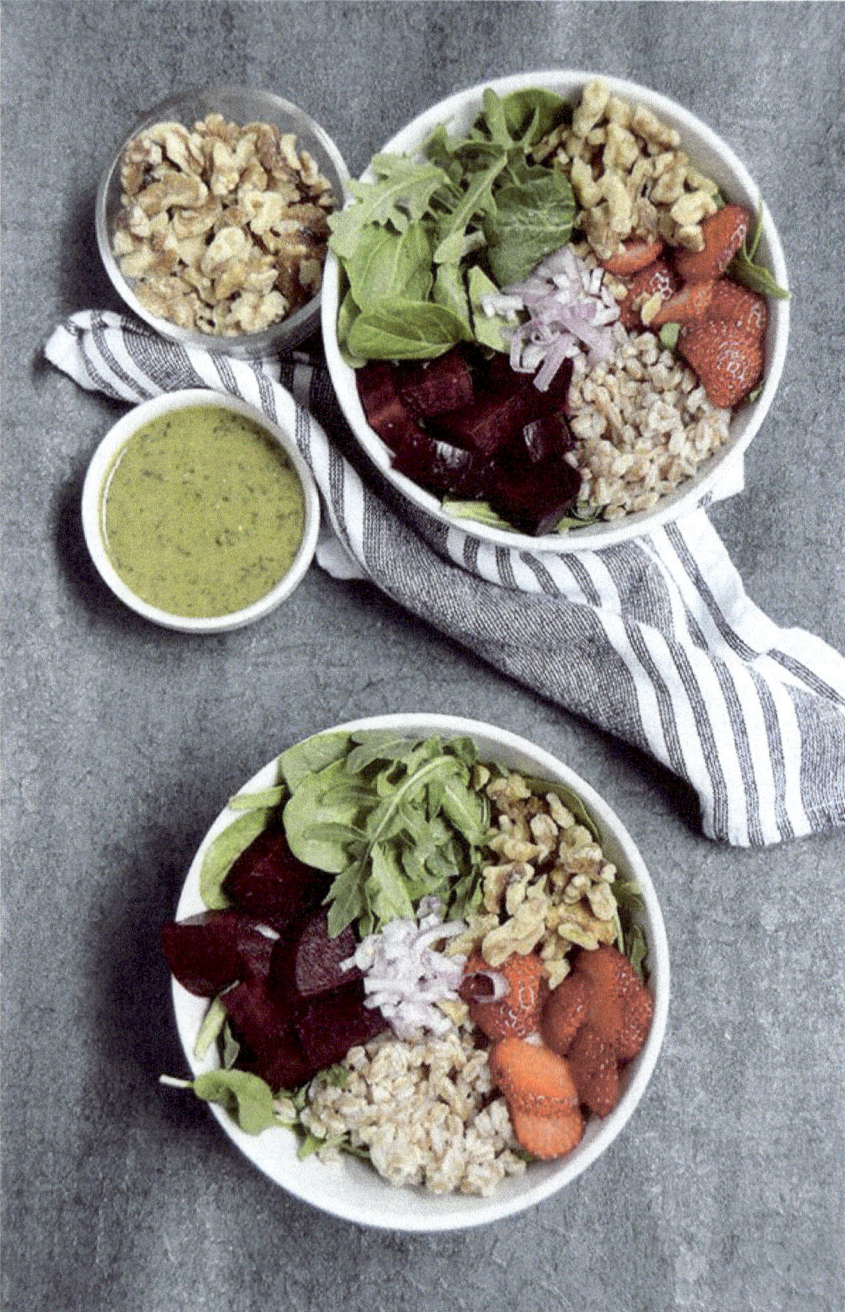

Preparation Time: 10 minutes

Cooking Time: 0 minutes

Servings: 4

Ingredients :

Ingredients for the dressing

- ¼ cup blackberries

- ¼ cup extra-virgin olive oil

- Juice of 1 lemon

- 2 tablespoons minced fresh basil

- 1 teaspoon poppy seeds

- A pinch of sea salt

- For the salad

- 2 celery stalks, chopped

- 4 cooked beets, peeled and chopped

- 1 cup blackberries

- 4 cups spring mix

Directions:

1. To make the dressing, mash the blackberries in a bowl. Whisk in the oil, lemon juice, basil, poppy seeds, and sea salt.

2. To make the salad: Add the celery, beets, blackberries, and spring mix to the bowl with the dressing.

3. Combine and serve.

Nutrition:

Calories: 192

Fat: 15g

Carbohydrates: 15g

Protein: 2g

Basic Salad With Olive Oil Dressing

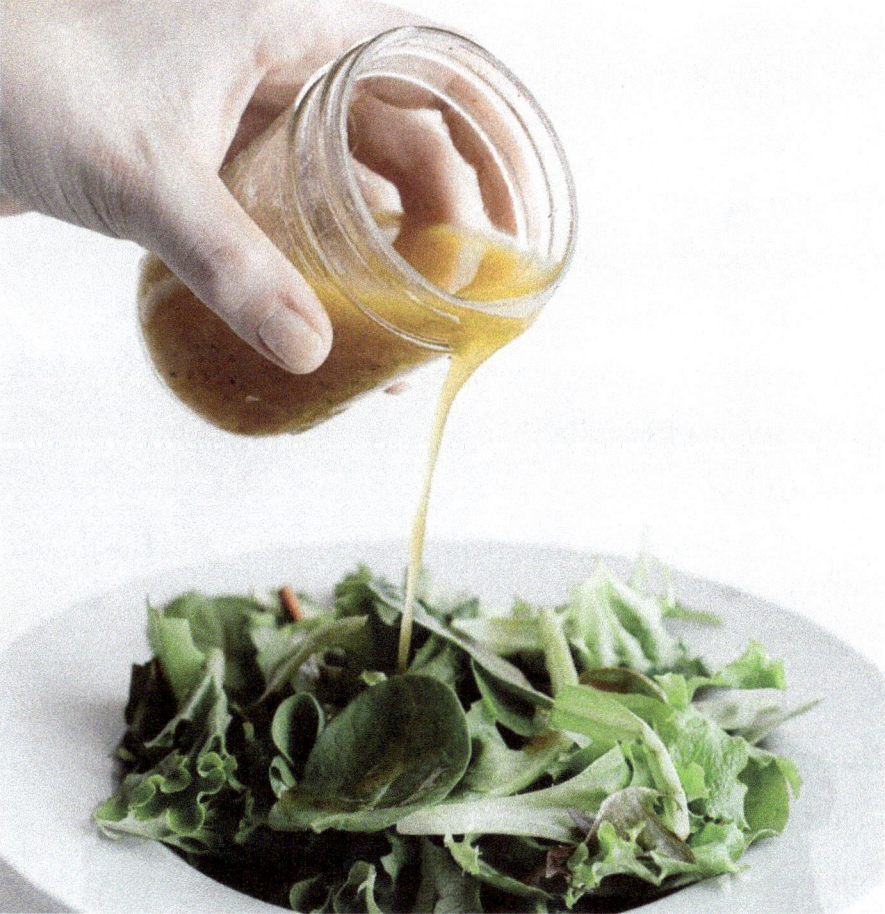

Preparation Time: 10 minutes

Cooking Time: 0 minute

Servings: 4

Ingredients :

- 1 cup coarsely chopped iceberg lettuce
- 1 cup coarsely chopped romaine lettuce
- 1 cup fresh baby spinach
- 1 large tomato, hulled and coarsely chopped
- 1 cup diced cucumber
- 2 tablespoons extra-virgin olive oil
- ¼ teaspoon of sea salt

Directions:

1. In a bowl, combine the spinach and lettuces. Add the tomato and cucumber.

2. Drizzle with oil and sprinkle with sea salt.

3. Mix and serve.

Nutrition:

Calories: 77

Fat: 4g

Carbohydrates: 3g

Protein: 1g

Spinach & Orange Salad With Oil Drizzle

Preparation Time: 10 minutes

Cooking Time: 0 minute

Servings: 4

Ingredients :

- 4 cups fresh baby spinach
- 1 blood orange, coarsely chopped
- ½ red onion, thinly sliced
- ½ shallot, finely chopped
- 2 tbsp. minced fennel fronds
- Juice of 1 lemon
- 1 tbsp. extra-virgin olive oil
- Pinch sea salt

Directions:

1. In a bowl, toss together the spinach, orange, red onion, shallot, and fennel fronds.

2. Add the lemon juice, oil, and sea salt.

3. Mix and serve.

Nutrition:

Calories: 79

Fat: 2g

Carbohydrates: 8g

Protein: 1g

Fruit Salad With Coconut-Lime Dressing

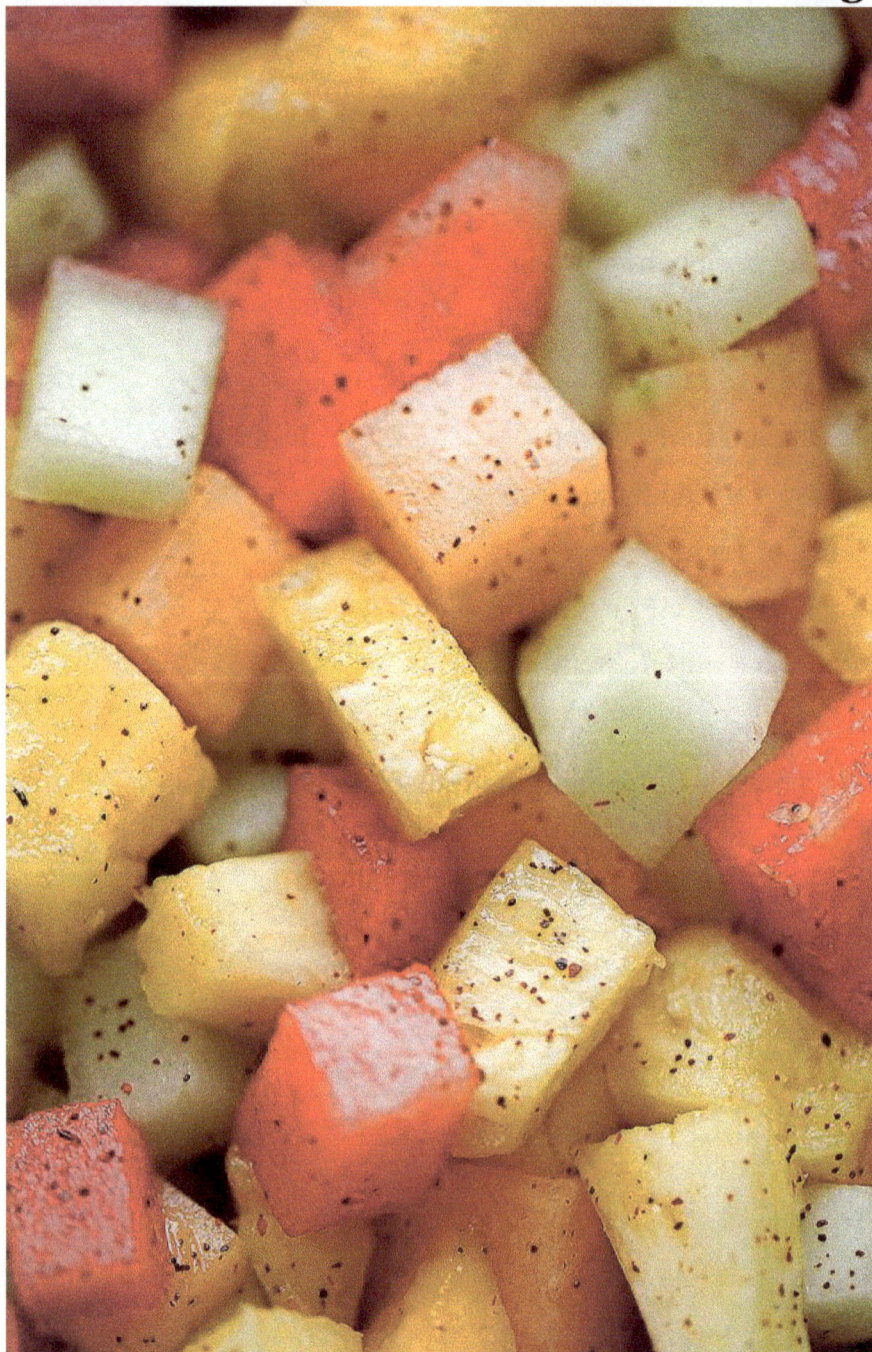

Preparation Time: 5 minutes

Cooking Time: 0 minutes

Servings: 4

Ingredients :

Ingredients for the dressing

- ¼ cup full-fat canned coconut milk
- 1 tbsp. raw honey
- Juice of ½ lime
- Pinch sea salt
- For the salad
- 2 bananas, thinly sliced
- 2 mandarin oranges, segmented
- ½ cup strawberries, thinly sliced
- ½ cup raspberries
- ½ cup blueberries

Directions:

1. To make the dressing: whisk all the dressing **Ingredients** in a bowl.

2. To make the salad: Add the salad Ingredients in a bowl and mix.

3. Drizzle with the dressing and serve.

Nutrition:

Calories: 141

Fat: 3g

Carbohydrates: 30g

Protein: 2g

Parsnip, Carrot, And Kale Salad With Dressing

Preparation Time: 10 minutes

Cooking Time: 0 minutes

Servings: 4

Ingredients :

Ingredients for the dressing

- ⅓ cup extra-virgin olive oil

- Juice of 1 lime

- 2 tbsp. minced fresh mint leaves

- 1 tsp. pure maple syrup

- Pinch sea salt

For the salad

- 1 bunch kale, chopped

- ½ parsnip, grated

- ½ carrot, grated

- 2 tbsp. sesame seeds

Directions:

1. To make the dressing, mix all the dressing Ingredients in a bowl.

2. To make the salad, add the kale to the dressing and massage the dressing into the kale for 1 minute.

3. Add the parsnip, carrot, and sesame seeds.

4. Combine and serve.

Nutrition:

Calories: 214

Fat: 2g

Carbohydrates: 12g

Protein: 2g

Tomato Toasts

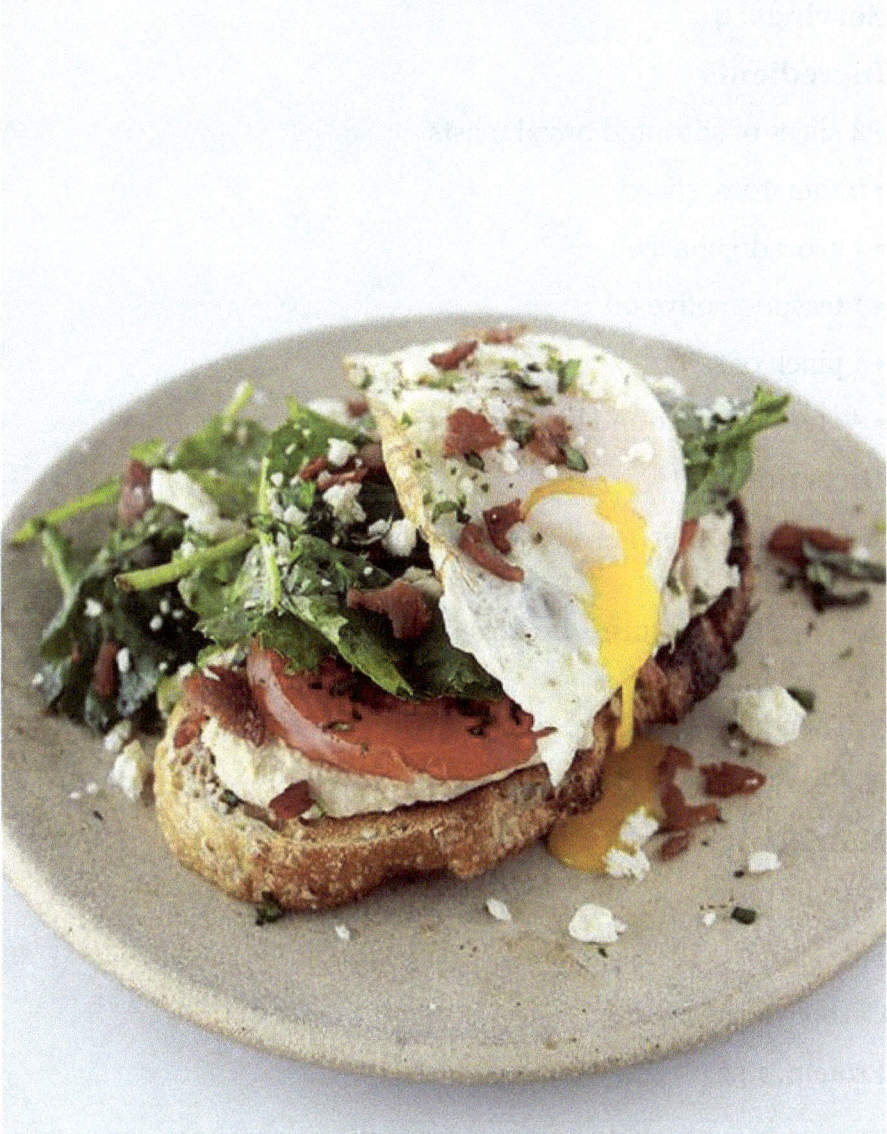

Preparation Time: 5 minutes

Cooking Time: 5 minutes

Servings: 4

Ingredients :

- 4 slices of sprouted bread toasts
- 2 tomatoes, sliced
- 1 avocado, mashed
- 1 teaspoon olive oil
- 1 pinch of salt
- ¾ teaspoon ground black pepper

Directions:

1. Blend together the olive oil, mashed avocado, salt, and ground black pepper.

2. When the mixture is homogenous – spread it over the sprouted bread.

3. Then place the sliced tomatoes over the toasts.

4. Enjoy!

Nutrition:

Calories: 125

Fat: 11.1g

Carbohydrates: 7.0g

Protein: 1.5g

Everyday Salad

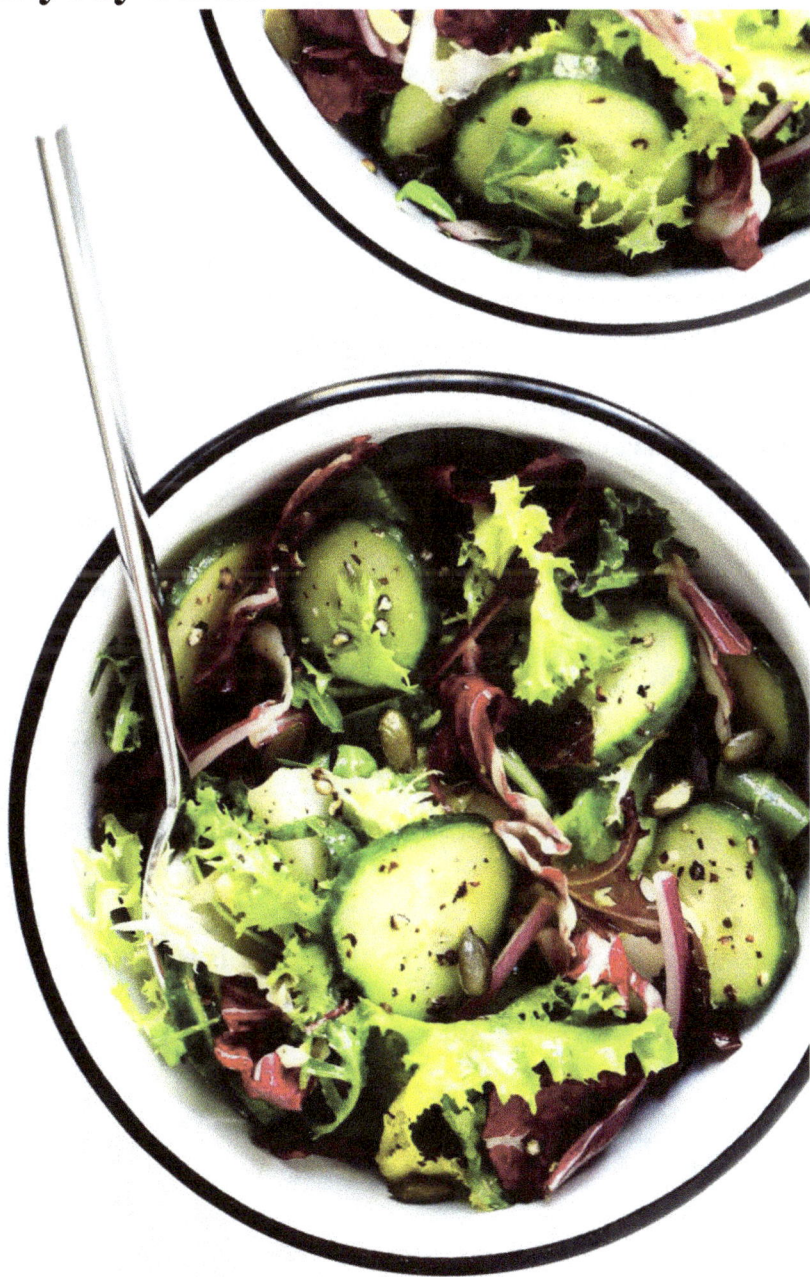

Preparation Time: 10 minutes

Cooking Time: 40 minutes

Servings: 6

Ingredients :

- 5 halved mushrooms
- 6 halved Cherry (Plum) Tomatoes
- 6 rinsed Lettuce Leaves
- 10 olives
- ½ chopped cucumber
- Juice from ½ Key Lime
- 1 teaspoon olive oil
- Pure Sea Salt

Directions:

1. Tear rinsed lettuce leaves into medium pieces and put them in a medium salad bowl.

2. Add mushrooms halves, chopped cucumber, olives and cherry tomato halves into the bowl. Mix well. Pour olive and Key Lime juice over salad.

3. Add pure sea salt to taste. Mix it all till it is well combined.

Nutrition:

Calories: 88

Carbohydrates: 11g

Fat: .5g

Protein: .8g

Super-Seedy Salad With Tahini Dressing

Preparation Time: 10 minutes

Cooking Time: 0 minutes

Servings: 1-2

Ingredients :

• 1 slice stale sourdough, torn into chunks

• 50g mixed seeds

• 1 tsp. cumin seeds

• 1 tsp. coriander seeds

• 50g baby kale

• 75g long-stemmed broccoli, blanched for a few minutes then roughly chopped

• ½ red onion, thinly sliced

• 100g cherry tomatoes, halved

• ½ a small bunch flat-leaf parsley, torn

DRESSING

• 100ml natural yogurt

• 1 tbsp. tahini

• 1 lemon, juiced

Directions:

1. Heat the oven to 200°C/fan 180°C/gas 6. Put the bread into a food processor and pulse into very rough breadcrumbs. Put into a bowl with the mixed seeds and spices, season, and spray well with oil. Tip onto a non-stick baking tray and roast for 15-20 minutes, stirring and tossing regularly, until deep golden brown.

2. Whisk together the dressing Ingredients, some seasoning and a splash of water in a large bowl. Tip the baby kale, broccoli, red onion, cherry tomatoes and flat-leaf parsley into the dressing, and mix well. Divide between 2 plates and top with the crispy breadcrumbs and seeds.

Nutrition:

Calories: 78

Carbohydrates: 6 g

Fat: 2g

Protein: 1.5g

Vegetable Salad

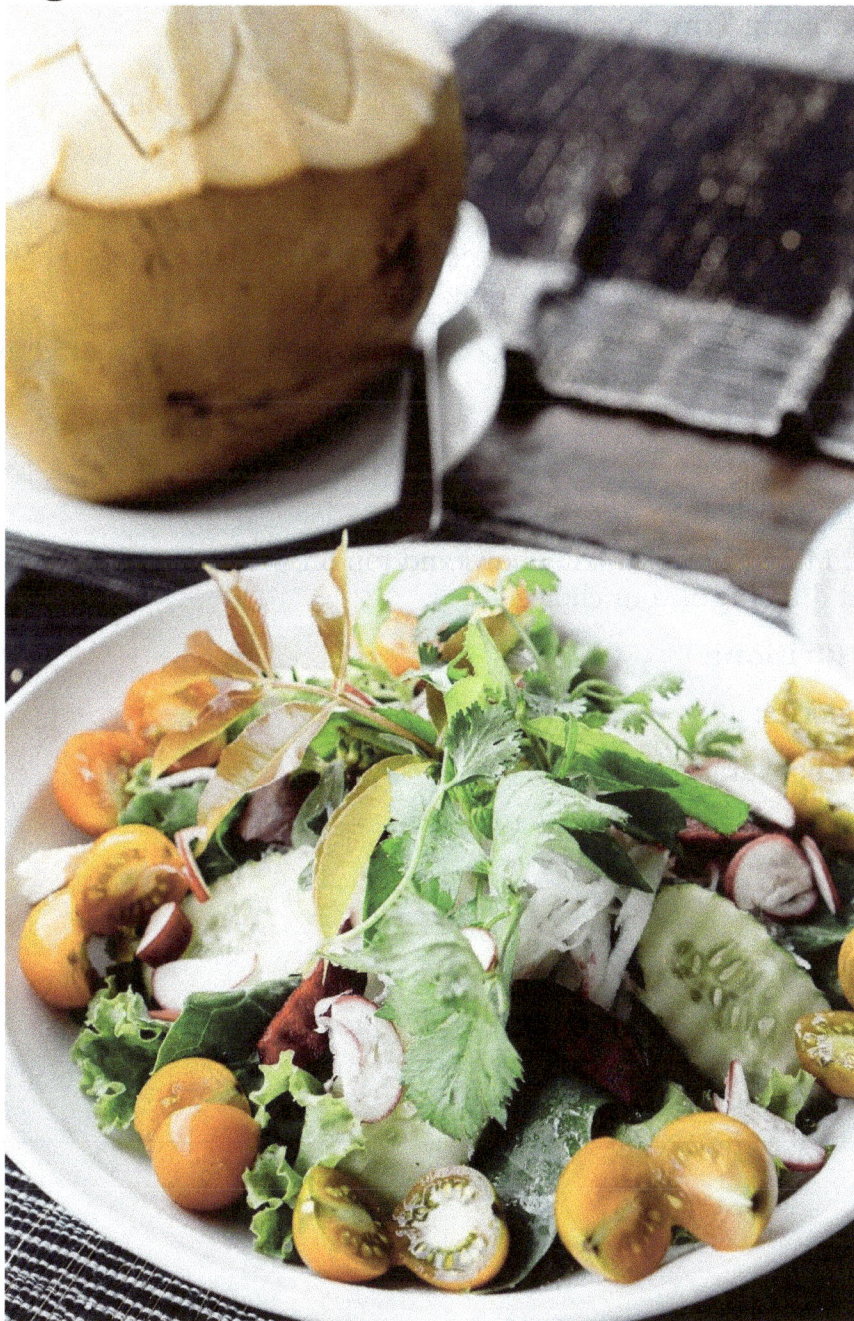

Preparation Time: 10 minutes

Cooking Time: 0 minutes

Servings: 1-2

Ingredients :

• 4 cups each of raw spinach and romaine lettuce

• 2 cups each of cherry tomatoes, sliced cucumber, chopped baby carrots and chopped red, orange and yellow bell pepper

• 1 cup each of chopped broccoli, sliced yellow squash, zucchini and cauliflower.

Directions:

3. Wash all these vegetables.

4. Mix in a large mixing bowl and top off with a non-fat or low-fat dressing of your choice.

Nutrition:

Calories: 48

Carbohydrates: 11g

Protein: 3g

Roasted Greek Salad

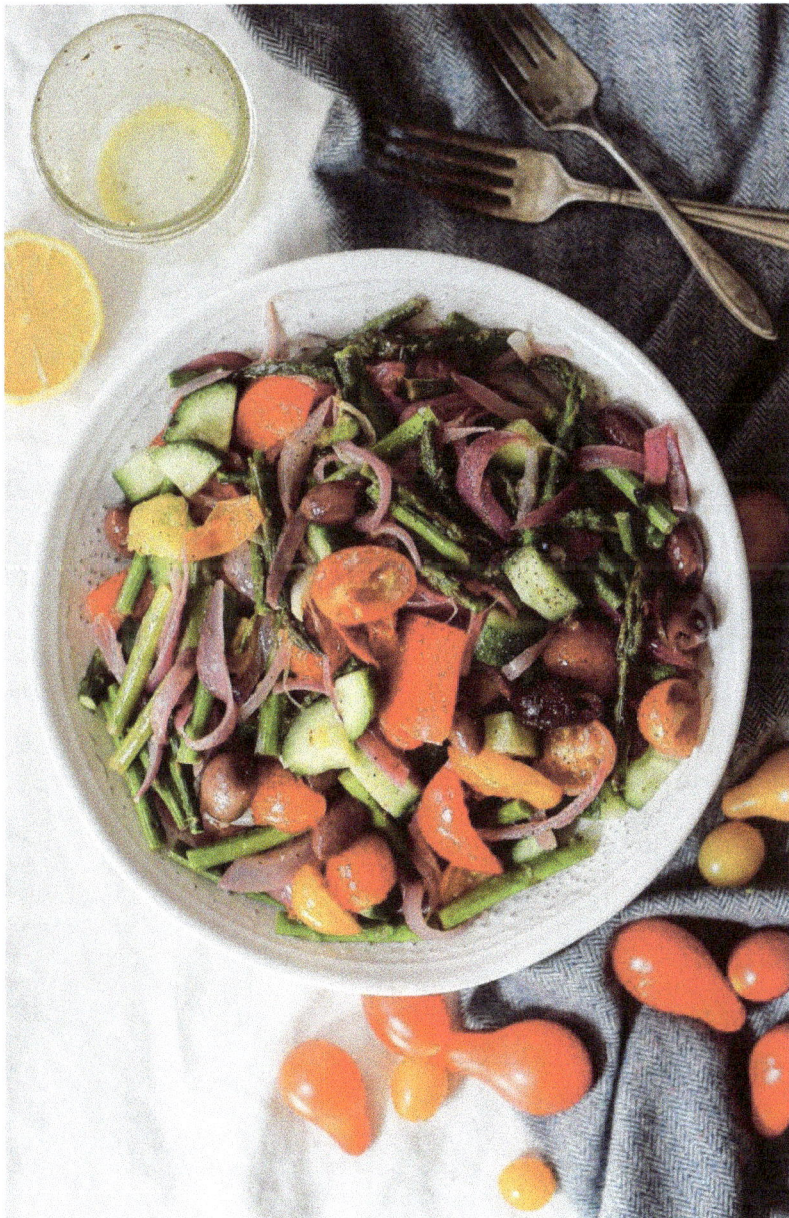

Preparation Time: 10 minutes

Cooking Time: 0 minutes

Servings: 1-2

Ingredients :

- 1 Romaine head, torn in bits
- 1 cucumber sliced
- 1 pint cherry tomatoes, halved
- 1 green pepper, thinly sliced
- 1 onion sliced into rings
- 1 cup kalamata olives
- 1 ½ cups feta cheese, crumbled
- For dressing combine:
- 1 cup olive oil
- 1/4 cup lemon juice
- 2 tsp. oregano
- Salt and pepper

Directions:

1. Lay Ingredients on plate.

2. Drizzle dressing over salad

Nutrition:

Calories: 107

Carbohydrates: 18g

Fat: 1.2 g

Protein: 1g

Alkaline Spring Salad

Preparation Time: 10 minutes

Cooking Time: 0 minutes

Servings: 1-2

Eating seasonal fruits and vegetables is a fabulous way of taking care of yourself and the environment at the same time. This alkaline-electric salad is delicious and nutritious.

Ingredients :

- 4 cups seasonal approved greens of your choice

- 1 cup cherry tomatoes

- 1/4 cup walnuts

- 1/4 cup approved herbs of your choice

- For the dressing:

- 3-4 key limes

- 1 tbsp. of homemade raw sesame

- Sea salt and cayenne pepper

Directions:

5. First, get the juice of the key limes. In a small bowl, whisk together the key lime juice with the homemade raw sesame "tahini" butter. Add sea salt and cayenne pepper, to taste.

6. Cut the cherry tomatoes in half.

7. In a large bowl, combine the greens, cherry tomatoes , and herbs. Pour the dressing on top and "massage" with your hands.

8. Let the greens soak up the dressing. Add more sea salt, cayenne pepper, and herbs on top if you wish. Enjoy!

Nutrition:

Calories: 77

Carbohydrates: 11g

Tuna Salad

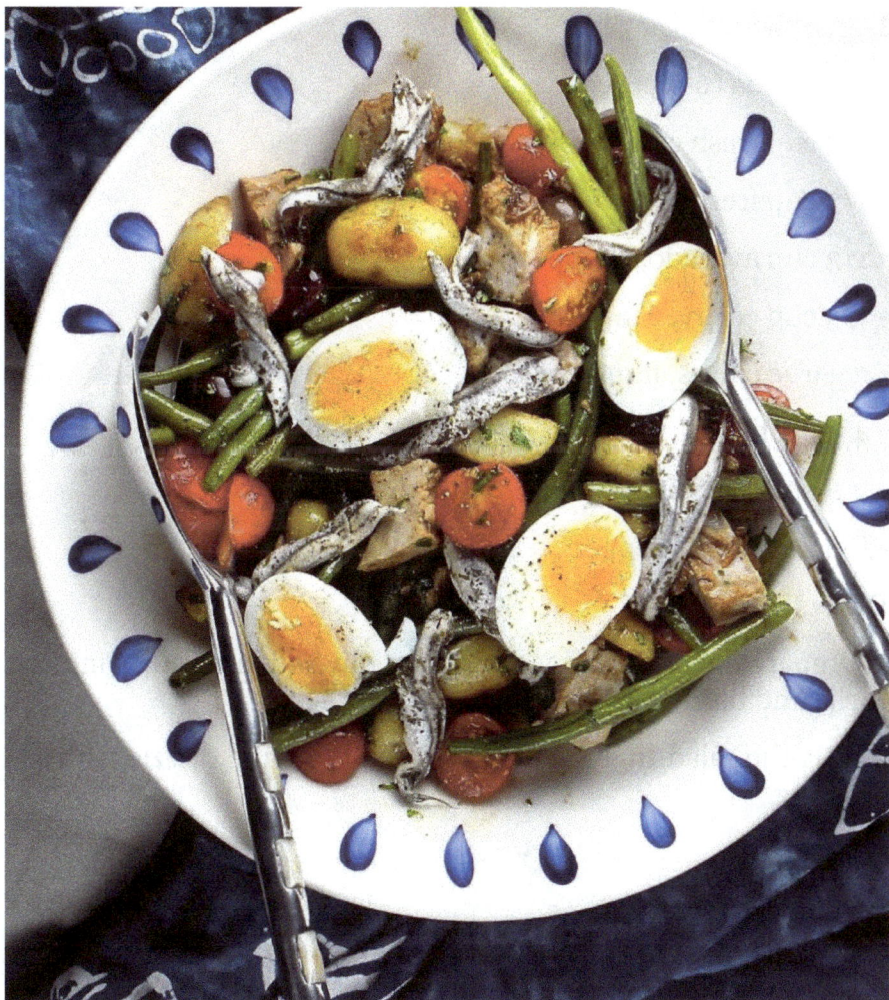

Preparation Time: 10 minutes

Cooking Time: none

Servings: 3

Ingredients :

- 1 can tuna (6 oz.)
- 1/3 cup fresh cucumber, chopped
- 1/3 cup fresh tomato, chopped
- 1/3 cup avocado, chopped
- 1/3 cup celery, chopped
- 2 garlic cloves, minced
- 4 tsp. olive oil
- 2 tbsp. lime juice
- Pinch of black pepper

Directions:

1. Prepare the dressing by combining olive oil, lime juice, minced garlic and black pepper.

2. Mix the salad Ingredients in a salad bowl and drizzle with the dressing.

Nutrition:

Carbohydrates: 4.8 g

Protein: 14.3 g

Total sugars: 1.1 g

Calories: 212 g

Roasted Portobello Salad

Preparation Time: 10 minutes

Cooking Time: none

Servings: 4

Ingredients :

- 11/2 lb. Portobello mushrooms, stems trimmed
- 3 heads Belgian endive, sliced
- 1 small red onion, sliced
- 4 oz. blue cheese
- 8 oz. mixed salad greens
- Dressing:
- 3 tbsp. red wine vinegar
- 1 tbsp. Dijon mustard
- Servings cup olive oil
- Salt and pepper to taste

Directions:

1. Preheat the oven to 450F.

2. Prepare the dressing by whisking together vinegar, mustard, salt and pepper. Slowly add olive oil while whisking.

3. Cut the mushrooms and arrange them on a baking sheet, stem-side up. Coat the mushrooms with some dressing and bake for 15 minutes.

4. In a salad bowl toss the salad greens with onion, endive and cheese. Sprinkle with the dressing.

5. Add mushrooms to the salad bowl.

Nutrition:

Carbohydrates: 22.3 g

Protein: 14.9 g

Total sugars: 2.1 g

Calories: 501

Shredded Chicken Salad

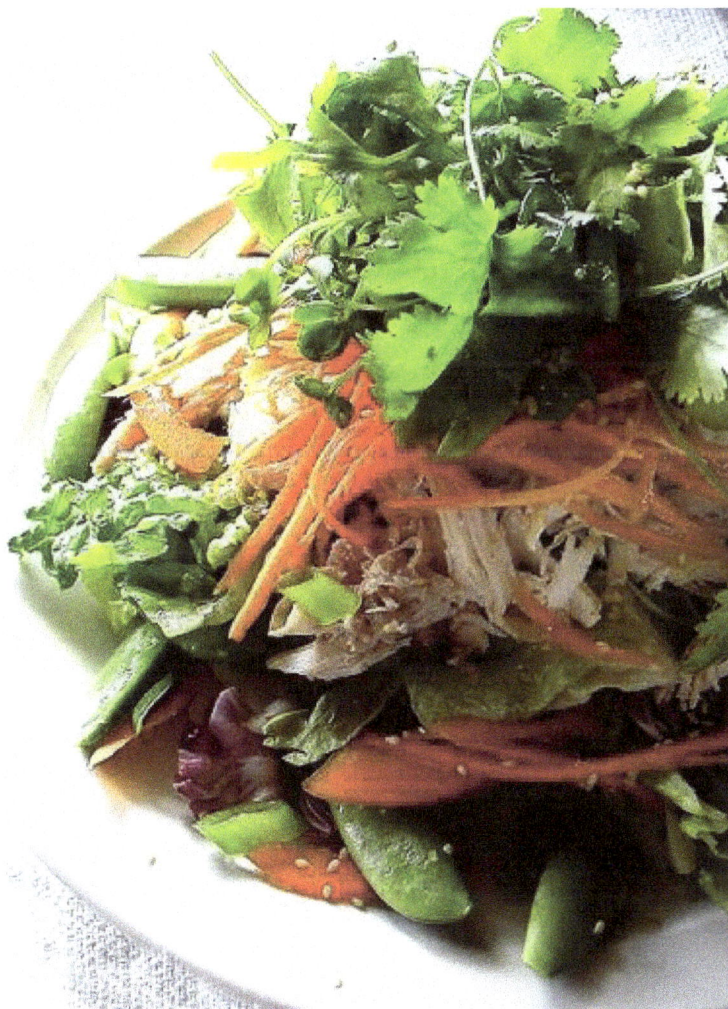

Preparation Time: 5 minutes

Cooking Time: 10 minutes

Servings: 6

Ingredients :

- 2 chicken breasts, boneless, skinless
- 1 head iceberg lettuce, cut into strips
- 2 bell peppers, cut into strips
- 1 fresh cucumber, quartered, sliced
- 3 scallions, sliced
- 2 tbsp. chopped peanuts
- 1 tbsp. peanut vinaigrette
- Salt to taste
- 1 cup water

Directions:

1. In a skillet simmer one cup of salted water.

2. Add the chicken breasts, cover and cook on low for 5 minutes. Remove the cover. Then remove the chicken from the skillet and shred with a fork.

3. In a salad bowl mix the vegetables with the cooled chicken, season with salt and sprinkle with peanut vinaigrette and chopped peanuts.

Nutrition:

Carbohydrates: 9 g

Protein: 11.6 g

Total sugars: 4.2 g

Calories: 117

Cherry Tomato Salad

Preparation Time: 10 minutes

Cooking Time: none

Servings: 6

Ingredients :

• 40 cherry tomatoes, halved

• 1 cup mozzarella balls, halved

• 1 cup green olives, sliced

• 1 can (6 oz.) black olives, sliced

• 2 green onions, chopped

• 3 oz. roasted pine nuts

• Dressing:

• 1/2 cup olive oil

• 2 tbsp. red wine vinegar

• 1 tsp. dried oregano

• Salt and pepper to taste

Directions:

1. In a salad bowl, combine the tomatoes, olives and onions.

2. Prepare the dressing by combining olive oil with red wine vinegar, dried oregano, salt and pepper.

3. Sprinkle with the dressing and add the nuts.

4. Let marinate in the fridge for 15 minutes.

Nutrition:

Carbohydrates: 10.7 g

Protein: 2.4 g

Total sugars: 3.6 g

Ground Turkey Salad

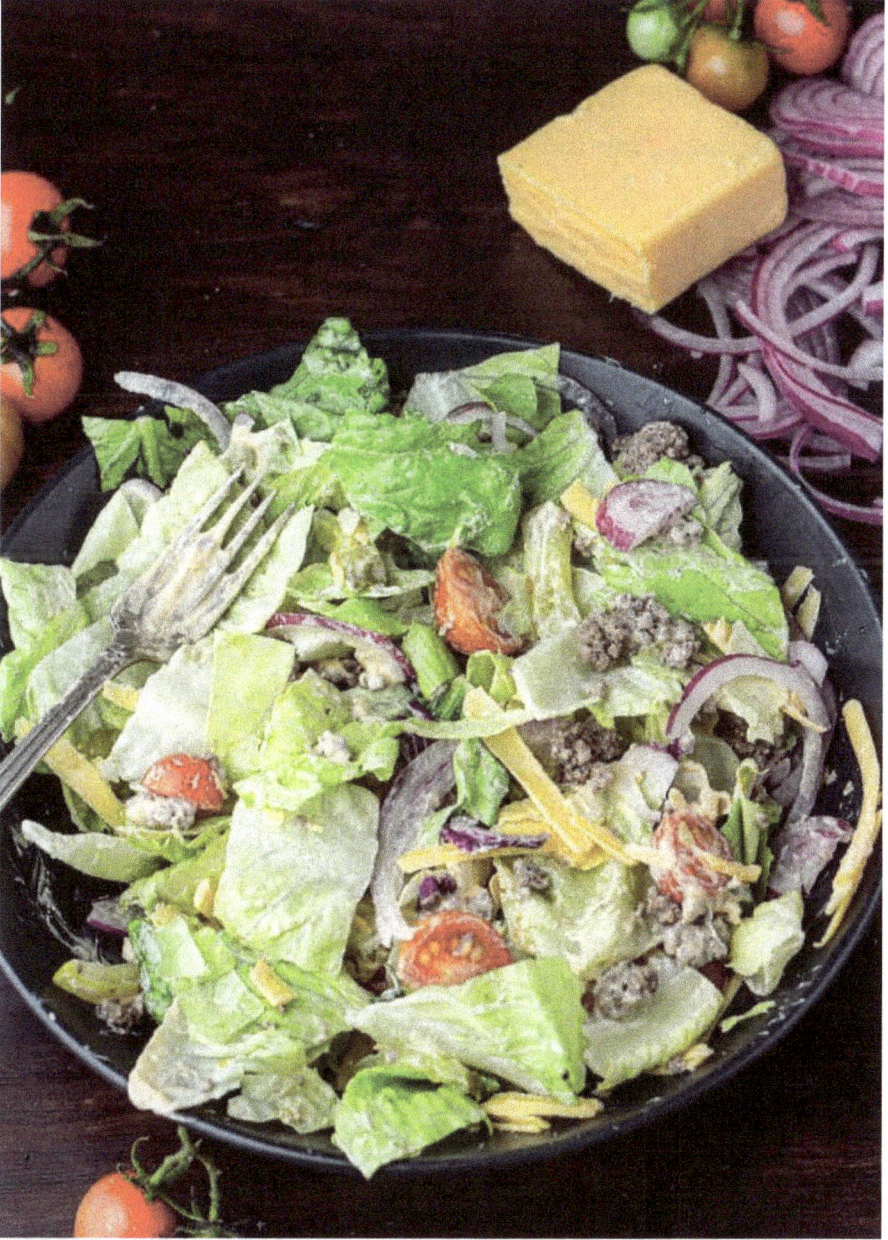

Preparation Time: 10 minutes

Cooking Time: 35 minutes

Servings: 6

Ingredients :

- 1 lb. lean ground turkey
- 1/2 inch ginger, minced
- 2 garlic cloves, minced
- 1 onion, chopped
- 1 tbsp. olive oil
- 1 bag lettuce leaves (for serving)
- ¼ cup fresh cilantro, chopped
- 2 tsp. coriander powder
- 1 tsp. red chili powder
- 1 tsp. turmeric powder
- Salt to taste
- 4 cups water
- Dressing:
- 2 tbsp. fat free yogurt
- 1 tbsp. sour cream, non-fat
- 1 tbsp. low fat mayonnaise
- 1 lemon, juiced
- 1 tsp. red chili flakes
- Salt and pepper to taste

Directions:

1. In a skillet sauté the garlic and ginger in olive oil for 1 minute. Add onion and season with salt. Cook for 10 minutes over medium heat.

2. Add the ground turkey and sauté for 3 more minutes. Add the spices (turmeric, red chili powder and coriander powder).

3. Add 4 cups water and cook for 30 minutes, covered.

4. Prepare the dressing by combining yogurt, sour cream, mayo, lemon juice, chili flakes, salt and pepper.

5. To serve arrange the salad leaves on serving plates and place the cooked ground turkey on them. Top with dressing.

Nutrition:

Carbohydrates: 9.1 g

Protein: 17.8 g

Total sugars: 2.5 g

Calories: 176

Asian Cucumber Salad

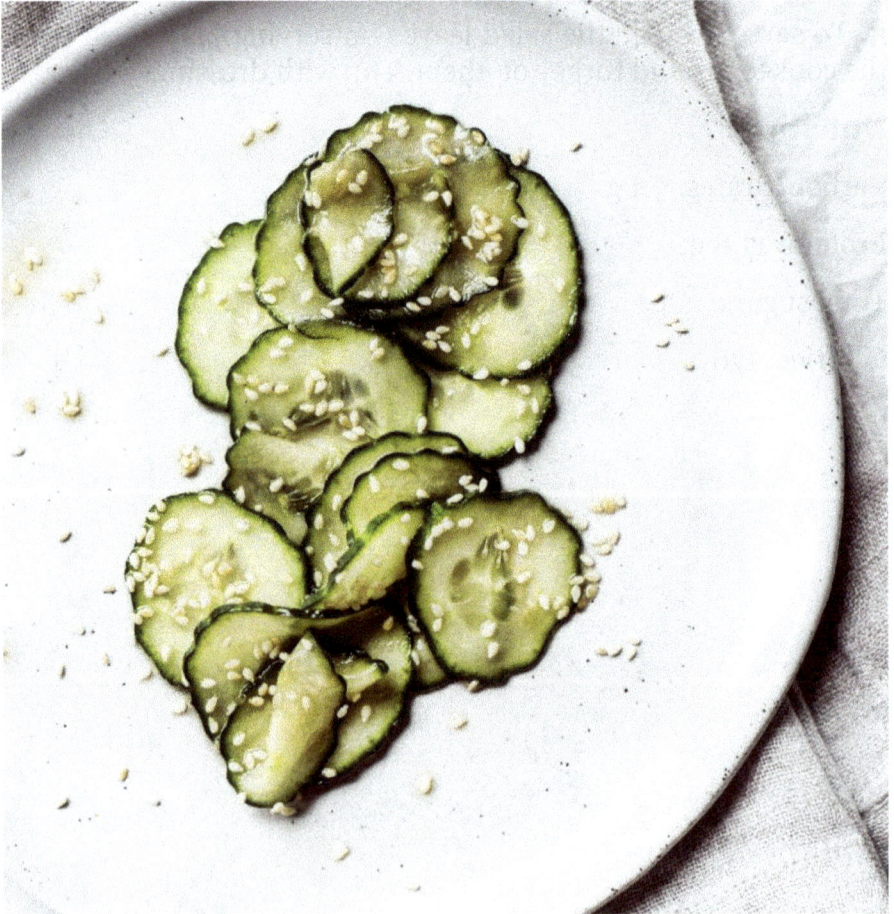

Preparation Time: 10 minutes

Cooking Time: none

Servings: 6

Ingredients :

- 1 lb. cucumbers, sliced

- 2 scallions, sliced

- 2 tbsp. sliced pickled ginger, chopped

- ¼ cup cilantro

- 1/2 red jalapeño, chopped

- 3 tbsp. rice wine vinegar

- 1 tbsp. sesame oil

- 1 tbsp. sesame seeds

Directions:

1. In a salad bowl combine all Ingredients and toss together.

Nutrition:

Carbohydrates: 5.7 g

Protein: 1 g

Total sugars: 3.1 g

Calories: 52

Cauliflower Tofu Salad

Preparation Time: 10 minutes

Cooking Time: 15 minutes

Servings: 4

Ingredients :

• 2 cups cauliflower florets, blended

• 1 fresh cucumber, diced

• 1/2 cup green olives, diced

• 1/3 cup red onion, diced

• 2 tbsp. toasted pine nuts

• 2 tbsp. raisins

• 1/3 cup feta, crumbled

• 1/2 cup pomegranate seeds

• 2 lemons (juiced, zest grated)

• 8 oz. tofu

• 2 tsp. oregano

• 2 garlic cloves, minced

• 1/2 tsp. red chili flakes

• 3 tbsp. olive oil

• Salt and pepper to taste

Directions:

1. Season the processed cauliflower with salt and transfer to a strainer to drain.

2. Prepare the marinade for tofu by combining 2 tbsp. lemon juice, 1.5 tbsp. olive oil, minced garlic, chili flakes, oregano, salt and pepper. Coat tofu in the marinade and set aside.

3. Preheat the oven to 450F.

4. Bake tofu on a baking sheet for 12 minutes.

5. In a salad bowl mix the remaining marinade with onions, cucumber, cauliflower, olives and raisins. Add in the remaining olive oil and grated lemon zest.

6. Top with tofu, pine nuts, and feta and pomegranate seeds.

Nutrition:

Carbohydrates: 34.1 g

Protein: 11.1 g

Total sugars: 11.5 g

Calories: 328

Scallop Caesar Salad

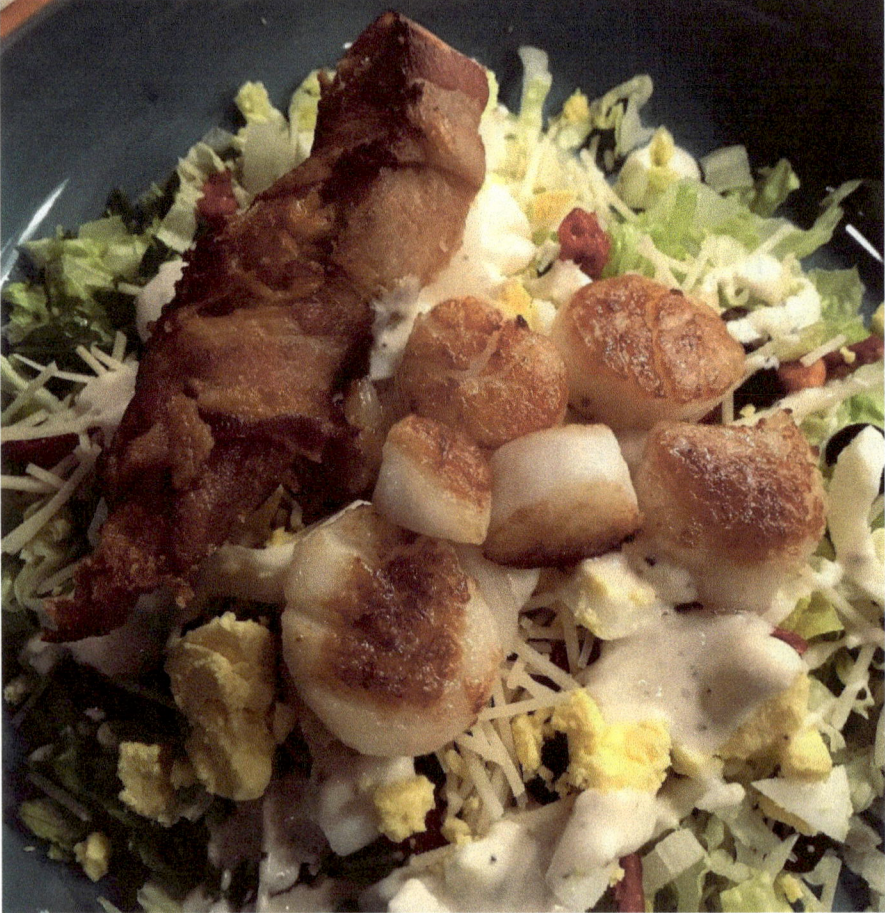

Preparation Time: 5 minutes

Cooking Time: 2 minutes

Servings: 2

Ingredients :

- 8 sea scallops
- 4 cups romaine lettuce
- 2 tsp. olive oil
- 3 tbsp. Caesar Salad Dressing
- 1 tsp. lemon juice
- Salt and pepper to taste

Directions:

1. In a frying pan heat olive oil and cook the scallops in one layer no longer than 2 minutes per both sides. Season with salt and pepper to taste.

2. Arrange lettuce on plates and place scallops on top.

3. Pour over the Caesar dressing and lemon juice.

Nutrition:

Carbohydrates: 14 g

Protein: 30.7 g

Total sugars: 2.2 g

Calories: 340 g

Chicken Avocado Salad

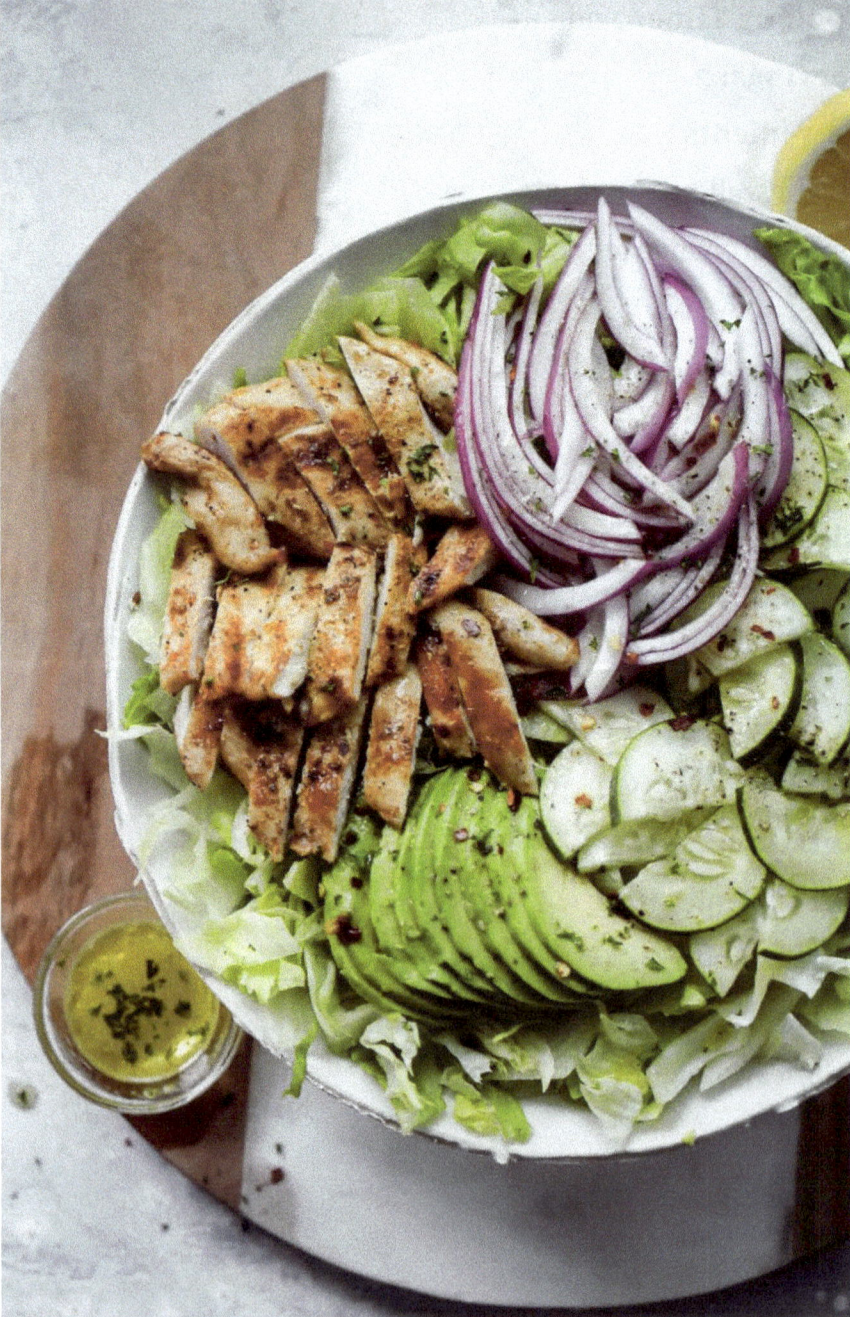

Preparation Time: 30 minutes

Cooking Time: 15 minutes

Servings: 4

Ingredients :

- 1 lb. chicken breast, cooked, shredded
- 1 avocado, pitted, peeled, sliced
- 2 tomatoes, diced
- 1 cucumber, peeled, sliced
- 1 head lettuce, chopped
- 3 tbsp. olive oil
- 2 tbsp. lime juice
- 1 tbsp. cilantro, chopped
- Salt and pepper to taste

Directions:

1. In a bowl whisk together oil, lime juice, cilantro, salt, and a pinch of pepper.

2. Combine lettuce, tomatoes, cucumber in a salad bowl and toss with half of the dressing.

3. Toss chicken with the remaining dressing and combine with vegetable mixture.

4. Top with avocado.

Nutrition:

Carbohydrates: 10 g

Protein: 38 g

Total sugars: 11.5 g

Calories: 380

California Wraps

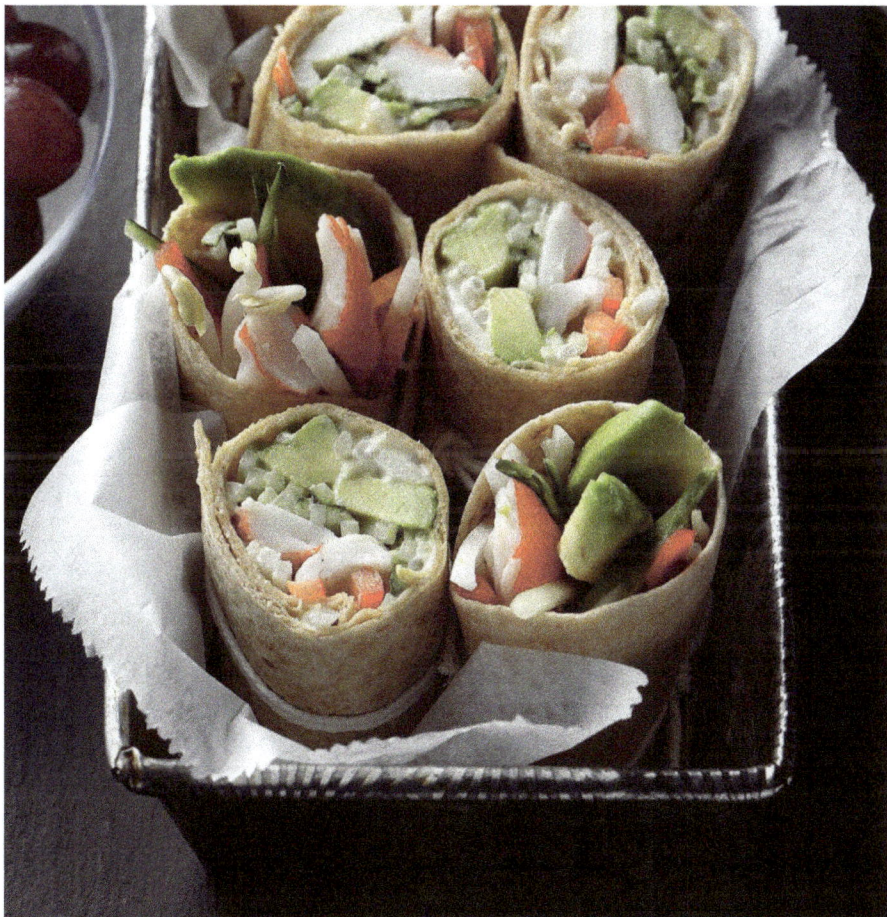

Preparation Time: 5 minutes

Cooking Time: 15 minutes

Servings: 4

Ingredients :

• 4 slices turkey breast, cooked

• 4 slices ham, cooked

• 4 lettuce leaves

• 4 slices tomato

• 4 slices avocado

• 1 tsp. lime juice

• A handful watercress leaves

• 4 tbsp. Ranch dressing, sugar free

Directions:

1. Top a lettuce leaf with turkey slice, ham slice and tomato.

2. In a bowl combine avocado and lime juice and place on top of tomatoes. Top with water cress and dressing.

3. Repeat with the remaining Ingredients for

4. Topping each lettuce leaf with a turkey slice, ham slice, tomato and dressing.

Nutrition:

Carbohydrates: 4 g

Protein: 9 g

Total sugars: 0.5 g

Calories: 14.

Chicken Salad In Cucumber Cups

Preparation Time: 5 minutes

Cooking Time: 15 minutes

Servings: 4

Ingredients :

• 1/2 chicken breast, skinless, boiled and shredded

• 2 long cucumbers, cut into 8 thick rounds each, scooped out (won't use in a).

• 1 tsp. ginger, minced

• 1 tsp. lime zest, grated

• 4 tsp. olive oil

• 1 tsp. sesame oil

• 1 tsp. lime juice

• Salt and pepper to taste

Directions:

1. In a bowl combine lime zest, juice, olive and sesame oils, ginger, and season with salt.

2. Toss the chicken with the dressing and fill the cucumber cups with the salad.

Nutrition:

Carbohydrates: 4 g

Protein: 12 g

Total sugars: 0.5 g

Calories: 116 g

Sunflower Seeds And Arugula Garden Salad

Preparation Time: 5 minutes

Cooking Time: 10 minutes

Servings: 6

Ingredients :

- ¼ tsp. black pepper
- ¼ tsp. salt
- 1 tsp. fresh thyme, chopped
- 2 tbsp. sunflower seeds, toasted
- 2 cups red grapes, halved
- 7 cups baby arugula, loosely packed
- 1 tbsp. coconut oil
- 2 tsp. honey
- 3 tbsp. red wine vinegar
- 1/2 tsp. stone-ground mustard

Directions:

1. In a small bowl, whisk together mustard, honey and vinegar. Slowly pour oil as you whisk.

2. In a large salad bowl, mix thyme, seeds, grapes and arugula.

3. Drizzle with dressing and serve.

Nutrition:

Calories: 86 7g

Protein: 1.6g

Carbs: 13.1g

Fat: 3.1g.

Supreme Caesar Salad

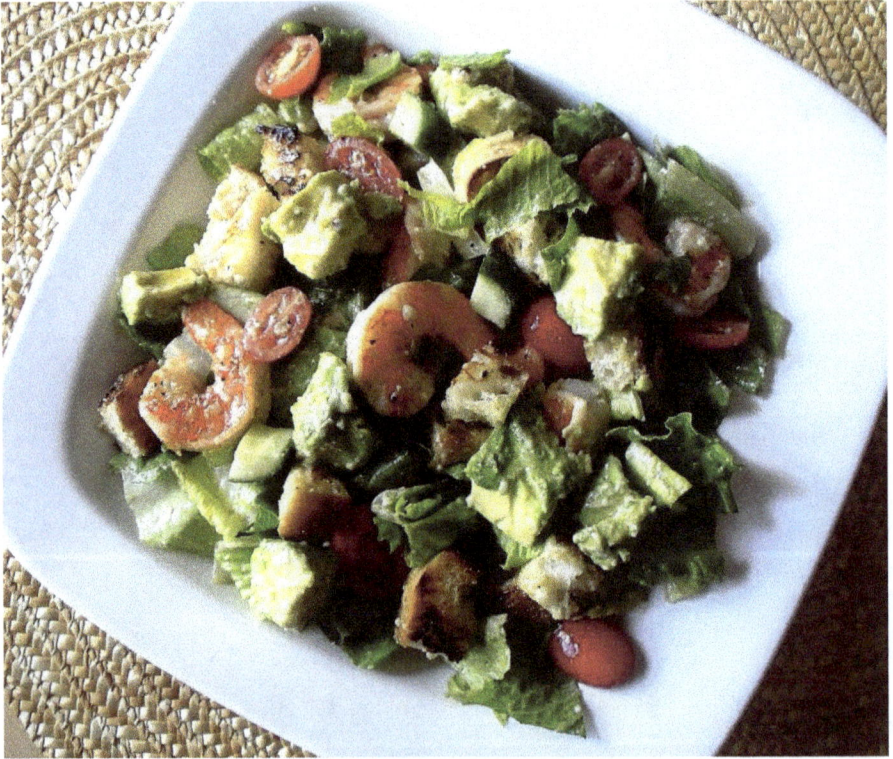

Preparation Time: 5 minutes

Cooking Time: 10 minutes

Servings: 4

Ingredients :

- ¼ cup olive oil
- ¾ cup mayonnaise
- 1 head romaine lettuce, torn into bite sized pieces
- 1 tbsp. lemon juice

- 1 tsp. Dijon mustard

- 1 tsp. Worcestershire sauce

- 3 cloves garlic, peeled and minced

- 3 cloves garlic, peeled and quartered

- 4 cups day old bread, cubed

- 5 anchovy filets, minced

- 6 tbsp. grated parmesan cheese, divided

- Ground black pepper to taste

- Salt to taste

Directions:

1. In a small bowl, whisk well lemon juice, mustard, Worcestershire sauce, 2 tbsp. parmesan cheese, anchovies, mayonnaise, and minced garlic. Season with pepper and salt to taste. Set aside in the ref.

2. On medium fire, place a large nonstick saucepan and heat oil.

3. Sauté quartered garlic until browned around a minute or two. Remove and discard.

4. Add bread cubes in same pan, sauté until lightly browned. Season with pepper and salt. Transfer to a plate.

5. In large bowl, place lettuce and pour in dressing. Toss well to coat. Top with remaining parmesan cheese.

6. Garnish with bread cubes, serve, and enjoy.

Nutrition:

Calories: 443.3g

Fat: 32.1g

Protein: 11.6g

Carbs: 27g

Tabbouleh- Arabian Salad

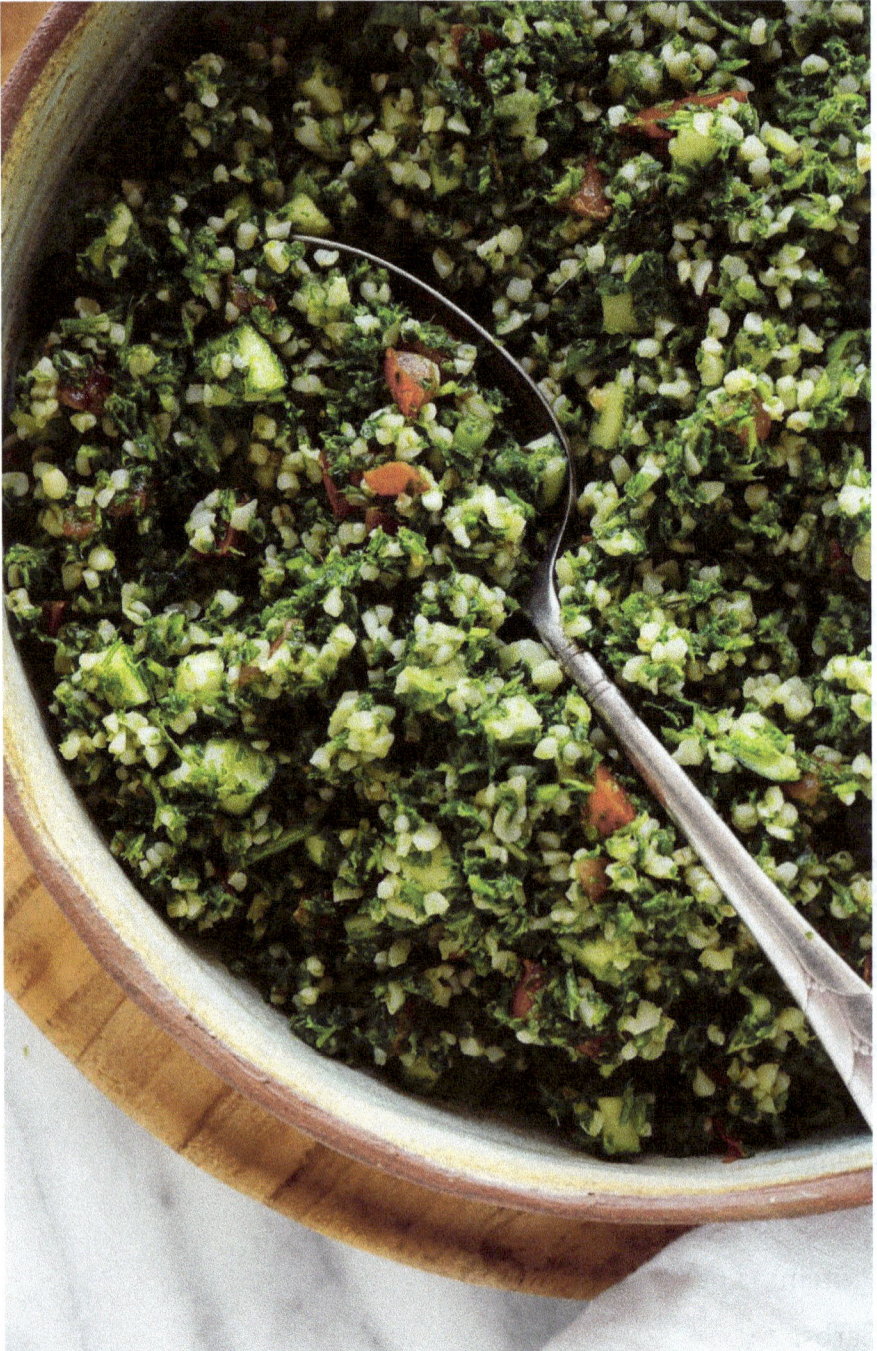

Preparation Time: 5 minutes

Cooking Time: 10 minutes

Servings: 6

Ingredients :

- ¼ cup chopped fresh mint
- 1 Servings: cups boiling water
- 1 cucumber, peeled, seeded and chopped
- 1 cup bulgur
- 1 cup chopped fresh parsley
- 1 cup chopped green onions
- 1 tsp. salt
- 1/3 cup lemon juice
- 1/3 cup olive oil
- 3 tomatoes, chopped
- Ground black pepper to taste

Directions:

1. In a large bowl, mix together boiling water and bulgur. Let soak and set aside for an while covered.

2. After 10 minutes, toss in cucumber, tomatoes, mint, parsley, onions, lemon juice and oil. Then season with black pepper and salt to taste. Toss well and refrigerate for another 20 minutes while covered before serving.

Nutrition:

Calories: 185.5g

fat: 13.1g

Protein: 4.1g

Carbs: 12.8g

Sarsaparilla Syrup

Preparation Time: 15 minutes

Cooking Time: 40 minutes

Servings: 4

Ingredients :

Date sugar, 1 c

Sassafras root, 1 tbsp.

Sarsaparilla root, 1 c

Water, 2 c

Directions:

1. Firstly add all of the Ingredients to a mason jar. Screw on the lid, tightly, and shake everything together. Heat a water bath up to 160. Sit the mason jar into the water bath and allow it to infuse for about 40 minutes.

2. When the infusion time is almost up, set up an ice bath. Add half and half water and ice to a bowl. Carefully take the mason jar out of the water bath and place it into the ice bath. Allow it to sit in the ice bath for 15 to 20 minutes.

3. Strain the infusion out and into another clean jar.

Nutrition:

Calories 37

Sugar 2g

Protein 0.4g

Fat 0.3

Dandelion "Coffee"

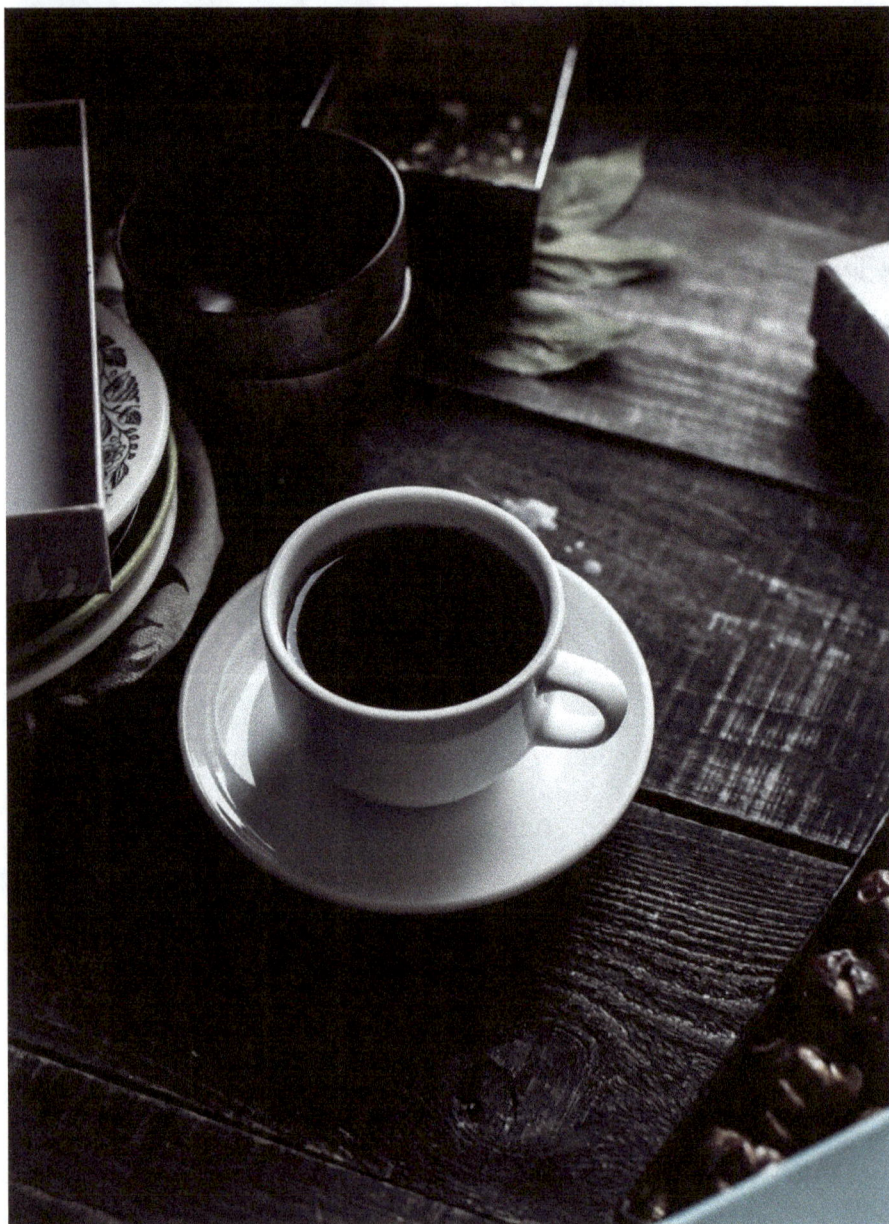

Preparation Time: 15 minutes

Cooking Time: 10 minutes

Servings: 4

Ingredients :

• Nettle leaf, a pinch

• Roasted dandelion root, 1 tbsp.

• Water, 24 oz.

Directions:

1. To start, we will roast the dandelion root to help bring out its flavors. Feel free to use raw dandelion root if you want to, but roasted root brings out an earthy and complex flavor, which is perfect for cool mornings.

2. Simply add the dandelion root to a pre-warmed cast iron skillet. Allow the pieces to roast on medium heat until they start to darken in color, and you start to smell their rich aroma. Make sure that you don't let them burn because this will ruin your teas taste.

3. As the root is roasting, have the water in a pot and allow it to come up to a full, rapid boil. Once your dandelion is roasted, add it to the boiling water with the nettle leaf. Steep this for ten minutes.

4. Strain. You can flavor your tea with some agave if you want to. Enjoy.

Nutrition:

Calories 43

Sugar 1g

Protein 0.2g

Fat 0.3

Chamomile Delight

Preparation Time: 5 minutes

Cooking Time: 10 minutes

Servings: 3

Ingredients :

• Date sugar, 1 tbsp.

• Walnut milk, .5 c

• 's Nerve/Stress Relief Herbal Tea, .25 c

• Burro banana, 1

Directions:

1. Prepare the tea according to the package Directions. Set to the side and allow to cool.

2. Once the tea is cooled, add it along with the above Ingredients to a blender and process until creamy and smooth.

Nutrition:

Calories 21

Sugar 0.8g

Protein 1.0g

Fat 0.2g

Mucus Cleanse Tea

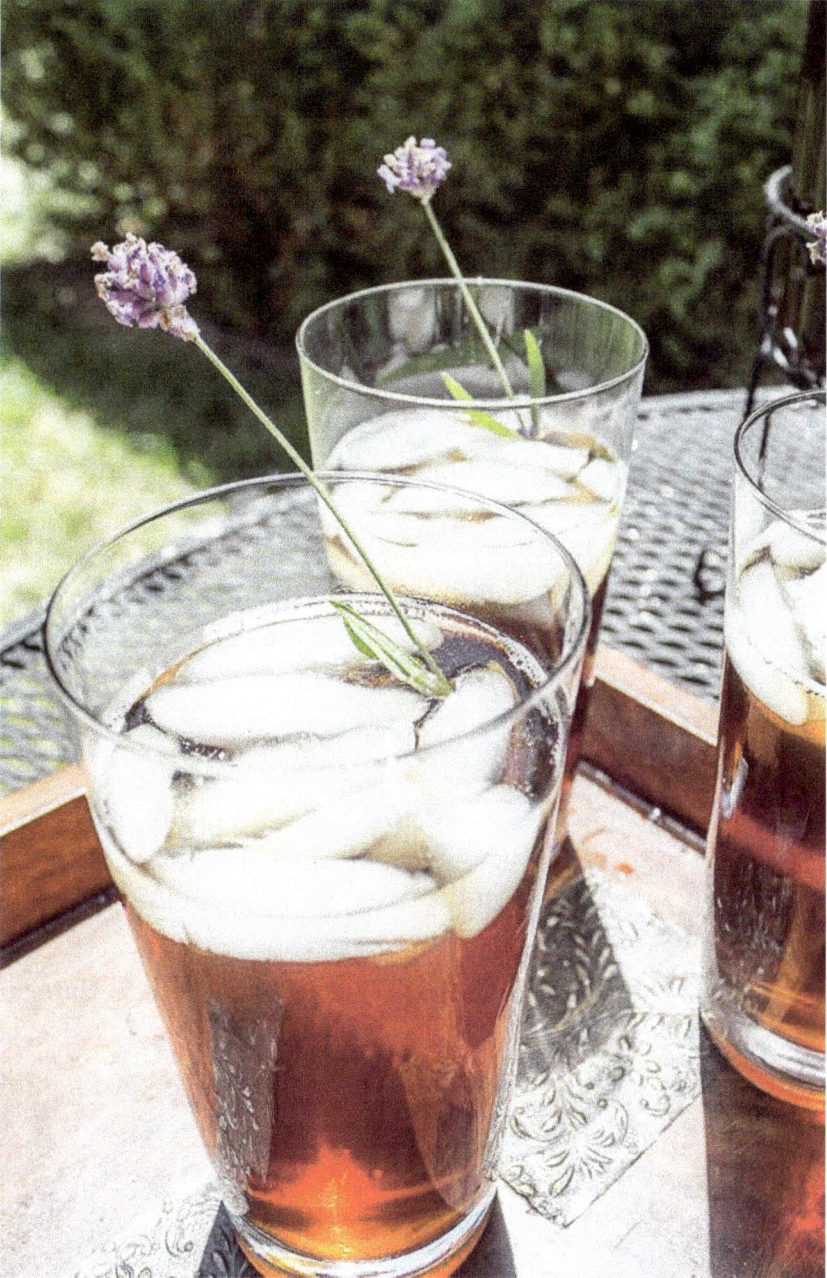

Preparation Time: 10 minutes

Cooking Time: 5 minutes

Servings: 2

Ingredients :

• Blue Vervain

• Bladder wrack

• Irish Sea Moss

Directions:

1. Add the sea moss to your blender. This would be best as a gel. Just make sure that it is totally dry.

2. Place equal parts of the bladder wrack to the blender. Again this would be best as a gel. Just make sure that it is totally dry. To get the best results you need to chop these by hand.

3. Add equal parts of the blue vervain to the blender. You can use the roots to increase your iron intake and Nutritional healing values.

4. Process the herbs until they form a powder. This can take up to three minutes.

5. Place the powder into a non-metal pot and put it on the stove. Fill the pot half full of water. Make sure the herbs are totally immersed in water. Turn on the heat and let the liquid boil. Don't let it boil more than five minutes.

6. Carefully strain out the herbs. You can save these for later use in other recipes.

7. You can add in some agave nectar, date sugar, or key lime juice for added flavor.

Nutrition:

Calories 36

Sugar 6g

Protein 0.7g

Fat 0.3g

Immune Tea

Preparation Time: 10 minutes

Cooking Time: 20 minutes

Servings: 1

Ingredients :

- Echinacea, 1 part
- Astragalus, 1 part
- Rosehip, 1 part
- Chamomile, 1 part
- Elderflowers, 1 part
- Elderberries, 1 part

Directions:

1. Mix the herbs together and place them inside an airtight container.

2. When you are ready to make a cup of tea, place one teaspoon into a tea ball or bag, and put it in eight ounces of boiling water. Let this sit for 20 minutes.

Nutrition:

Calories 39

Sugar 1g

Protein 2g

Fat 0.6g

Ginger Turmeric Tea

Preparation Time: 5 minutes

Cooking Time: 15 minutes

Servings: 2

Ingredients :

• Juice of one key lime

• Turmeric finger, couple of slices

• Ginger root, couple of slices

• Water, 3 c

Directions:

1. Pour the water into a pot and let it boil. Remove from heat and put the turmeric and ginger in. Stir well. Place lid on pot and let it sit 15 minutes.

2. While you are waiting on your tea to finish steeping, juice one key lime, and divide between two mugs.

3. Once the tea is ready, remove the turmeric and ginger and pour the tea into mugs and enjoy. If you want your tea a bit sweet, add some agave syrup or date sugar.

Nutrition:

Calories 27

Sugar 5g

Protein 3g

Fat 1.0g

Tranquil Tea

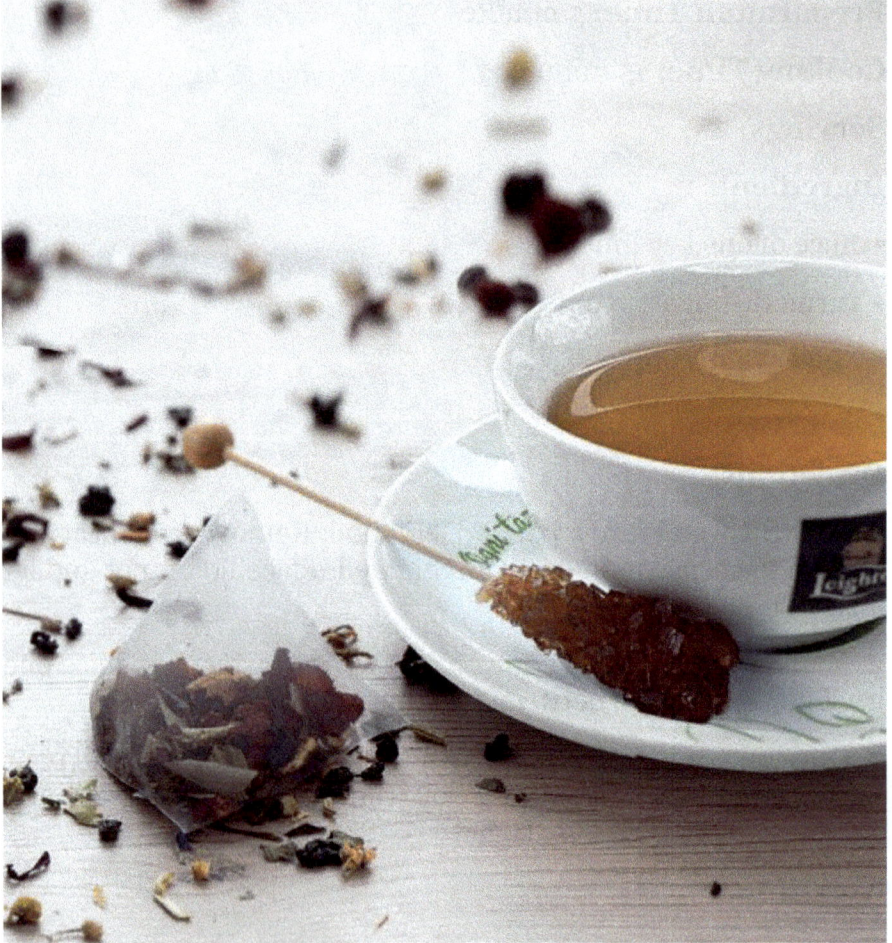

Preparation Time: 5 minutes

Cooking Time: 10 minutes

Servings: 2

Ingredients :

• Rose petals, 2 parts

• Lemongrass, 2 parts

• Chamomile, 4 parts

Directions:

1. Pour all the herbs into a glass jar and shake well to mix.

2. When you are ready to make a cup of tea, add one teaspoon of the mixture for every serving to a tea strainer, ball, or bag. Cover with water that has boiled and let it sit for ten minutes.

3. If you like a little sweetness in your tea, you can add some agave syrup or date sugar.

Nutrition:

Calories 35

Sugar 3.4g

Protein 2.3g

Fat 1.5g

Energizing Lemon Tea

Preparation Time: 5 minutes

Cooking Time: 15 minutes

Servings: 3

Ingredients :

• Lemongrass, .5 tsp. dried herb

• Lemon thyme, .5 tsp. dried herb

• Lemon verbena, 1 tsp. dried herb

Directions:

1. Place the dried herbs into a tea strainer, bag, or ball and place it in one cup of water that has boiled. Let this sit 15 minutes. Carefully strain out the tea. You can add agave syrup or date sugar if needed.

Nutrition:

Calories 40

Sugar 6g

Protein 2.2g

Fat 0.3

Respiratory Support Tea

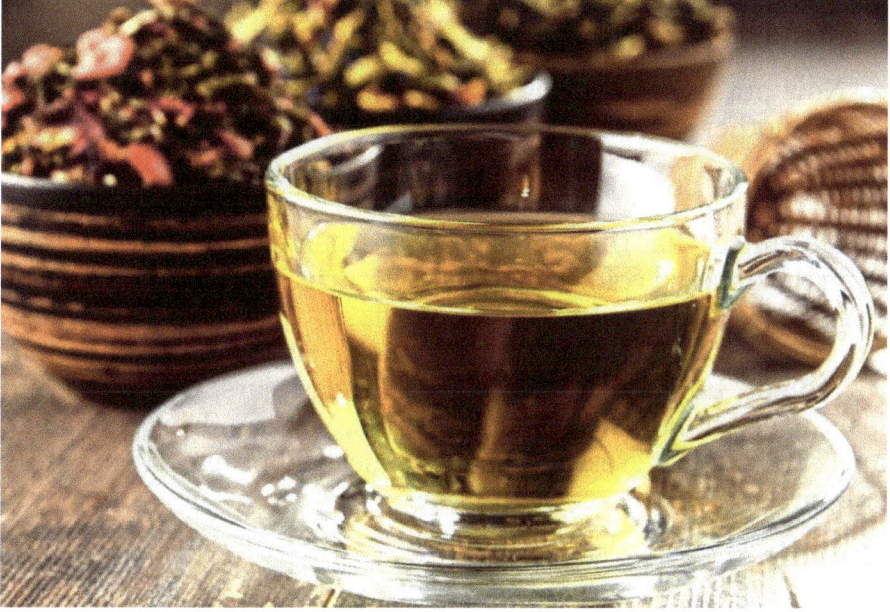

Preparation Time: 5 minutes

Cooking Time: 18 minutes

Servings: 4

Ingredients :

• Rosehip, 2 parts

• Lemon balm, 1 part

• Coltsfoot leaves, 1 part

• Mullein, 1 part

• Osha root, 1 part

• Marshmallow root, 1 part

Directions:

1. Place three cups of water into a pot. Place the Osha root and marshmallow root into the pot. Allow to boil. Let this simmer for ten minutes

2. Now put the remaining Ingredients into the pot and let this steep another eight minutes. Strain.

3. Drink four cups of this tea each day.

4. It's almost that time of year again when everyone is suffering from the dreaded cold. Then that cold turns into a nasty lingering cough. Having these Ingredients on hand will help you be able to get ahead of this year's cold season. When you buy your ingredient, they need to be stored in glass jars. The roots and leaves need to be put into separate jars. You can drink this tea at any time, but it is great for when you need some extra respiratory support.

Nutrition:

Calories 35

Sugar 3.4g

Protein 2.3g

Fat 1.5g

Thyme And Lemon Tea

Preparation Time: 5 minutes

Cooking Time: 10 minutes

Servings: 2

Ingredients :

• Key lime juice, 2 tsp.

• Fresh thyme sprigs, 2

Directions:

1. Place the thyme into a canning jar. Boil enough water to cover the thyme sprigs. Cover the jar with a lid and leave it alone for ten minutes. Add the key lime juice. Carefully strain into a mug and add some agave nectar if desired.

Nutrition:

Calories 22

Sugar 1.4g

Protein 5.3g

Fat 0.6g

Sore Throat Tea

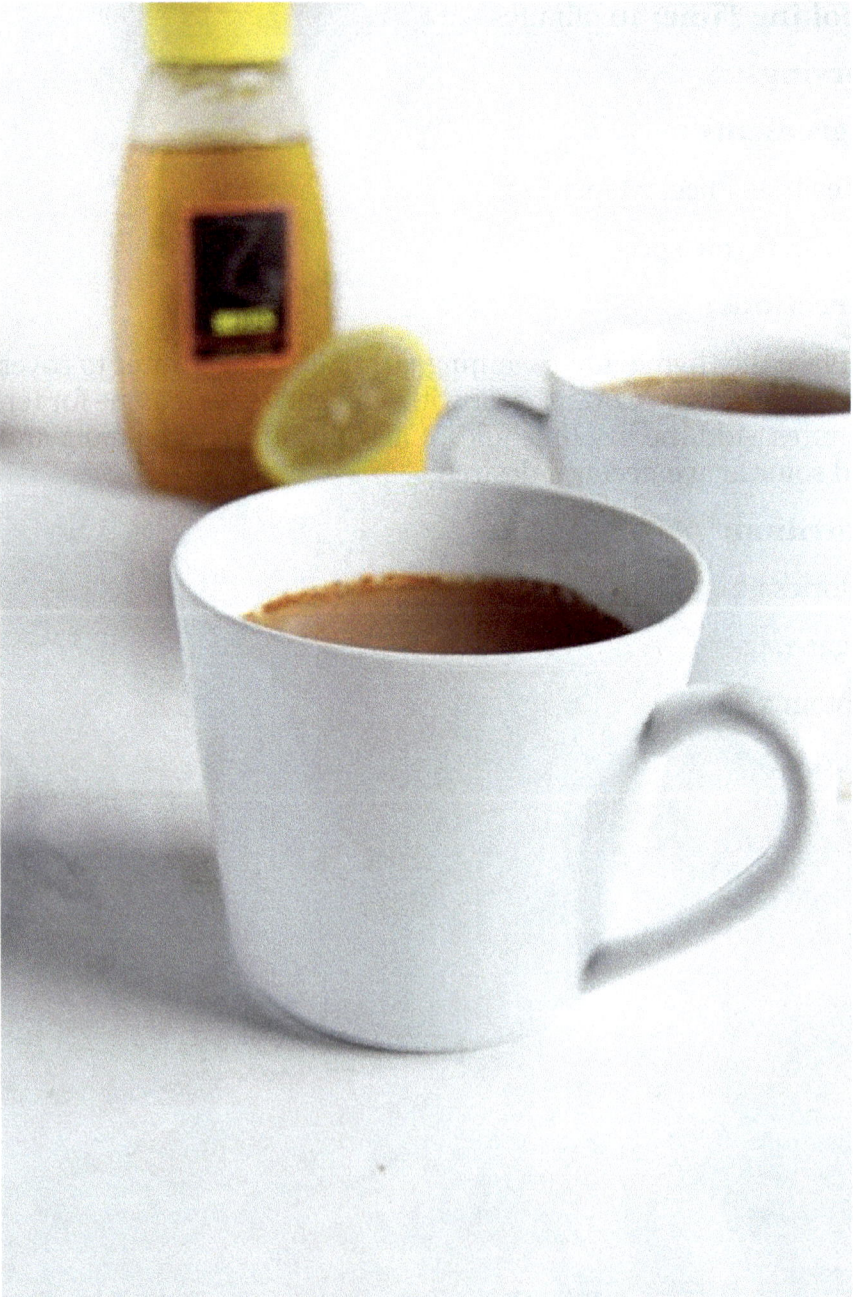

Preparation Time: 8 minutes

Cooking Time: 15 minutes

Servings: 4

Ingredients :

• Sage leaves, 8 to 10 leaves

Directions:

1. Place the sage leaves into a quart canning jar and add water that has boiled until it covers the leaves. Pour the lid on the jar and let sit for 15 minutes.

2. You can use this tea as a gargle to help ease a sore or scratchy throat. Usually, the pain will ease up before you even finish your first cup. This can also be used for inflammations of the throat, tonsils, and mouth since the mucous membranes get soothed by the sage oil. A normal dose would be between three to four cups each day. Every time you take a sip, roll it around in your mouth before swallowing it.

Nutrition:

Calories 26

Sugar 2.0g

Protein 7.6g

Fat 3.2g

Autumn Tonic Tea

Preparation Time: 10 minutes

Cooking Time: 15 minutes

Servings: 2

Ingredients :

- Dried ginger root, 1 part
- Rosehip, 1 part
- Red clover, 2 parts
- Dandelion root and leaf, 2 parts
- Mullein leaf, 2 parts
- Lemon balm, 3 parts
- Nettle leaf, 4 parts

Directions:

1. Place all of these Ingredients above into a bowl. Stir everything together to mix well. Put into a glass jar with a lid and keep it in a dry place that stays cool.

2. When you want a cup of tea, place four cups of water into a pot. Let this come to a full rolling boil. Place the desired amount of tea blend into a tea strainer, ball, or bag and cover with boiling water. Let sit for 15 minutes. Strain out the herbs and drink it either cold or hot. If you like your tea sweet, add some agave syrup or date sugar.

Nutrition:

Calories 43

Sugar 3.8g

Protein 6.5g

Fat 3.9g

Adrenal And Stress Health

Preparation Time: 12 minutes

Cooking Time: 20 minutes

Servings: 2

Ingredients :

Bladder wrack, .5 c

Tulsi holy basil, 1 c

Shatavari root, 1 c

Ashwagandha root, 1 c

Directions:

1. Place these Ingredients into a bowl. Stir well to combine.

2. Place mixture in a glass jar with a lid and store in a dry place that stays cool.

3. When you want a cup of tea, place two tablespoons of the tea mixture into a medium pot. Pour in two cups of water. Let this come to a full rolling boil. Turn down heat. Let this simmer 20 minutes. Strain well. If you prefer your tea sweet, you can add some agave syrup or date sugar.

Nutrition:

Calories 43

Sugar 2.2g

Protein 4.1g

Fat 2.3g

Lavender Tea

Preparation Time: 5 minutes

Cooking Time: 15 minutes

Servings: 2

Ingredients :

• Agave syrup, to taste

• Dried lavender flowers, 2 tbsp.

• Fresh lemon balm, handful

• Water, 3 c

Directions:

1. Pour the water in a pot and allow to boil.

2. Pour over the lavender and lemon balm. Cover and let sit for five minutes.

3. Strain well. If you prefer your tea sweet, add some agave syrup.

Nutrition:

Calories 59

Sugar 6.8g

Protein 3.3g

Fat 1.6g

Choco-Nut Milkshake

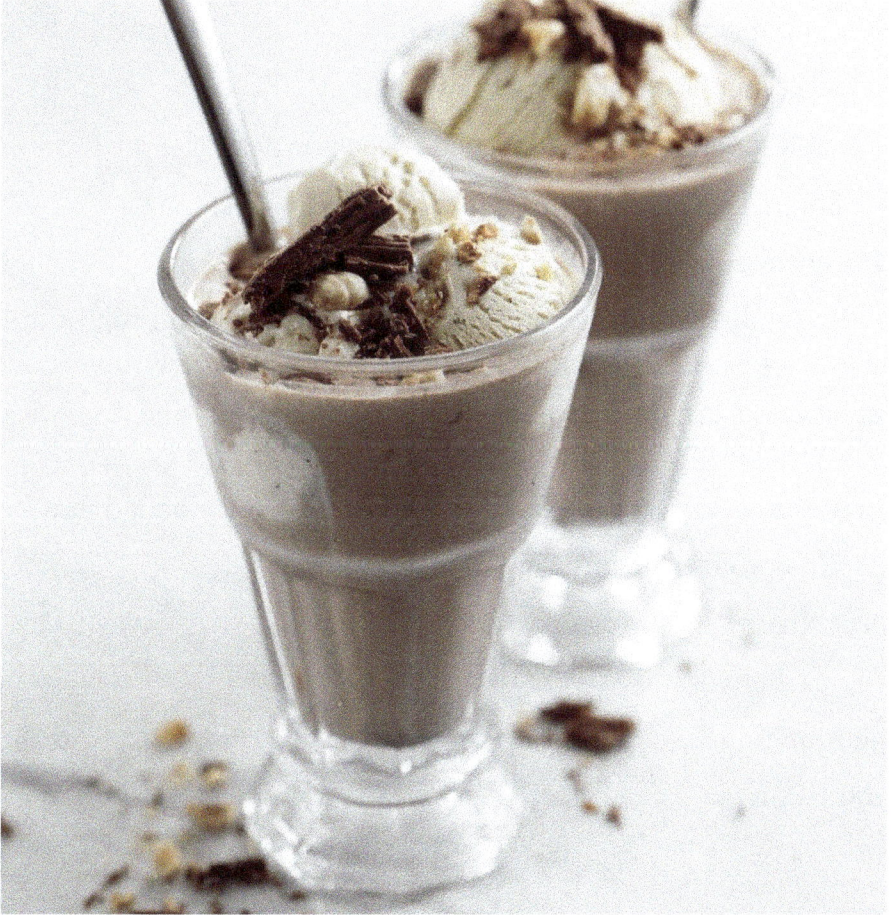

Preparation Time: 10 minutes

Cooking Time: 0 minute

Servings: 2

Ingredients

• 2 cups unsweetened coconut, almond

- 1 banana, sliced and frozen
- ¼ cup unsweetened coconut flakes
- 1 cup ice cubes
- ¼ cup macadamia nuts, chopped
- 3 tablespoons sugar-free sweetener
- 2 tablespoons raw unsweetened cocoa powder
- Whipped coconut cream

Directions:

1. Place all Ingredients into a blender and blend on high until smooth and creamy.

2. Divide evenly between 4 "mocktail" glasses and top with whipped coconut cream, if desired.

3. Add a cocktail umbrella and toasted coconut for added flair.

4. Enjoy your delicious Choco-nut smoothie!

Nutrition:

12g Carbohydrates

3g Protein

199 Calories

Pineapple & Strawberry Smoothie

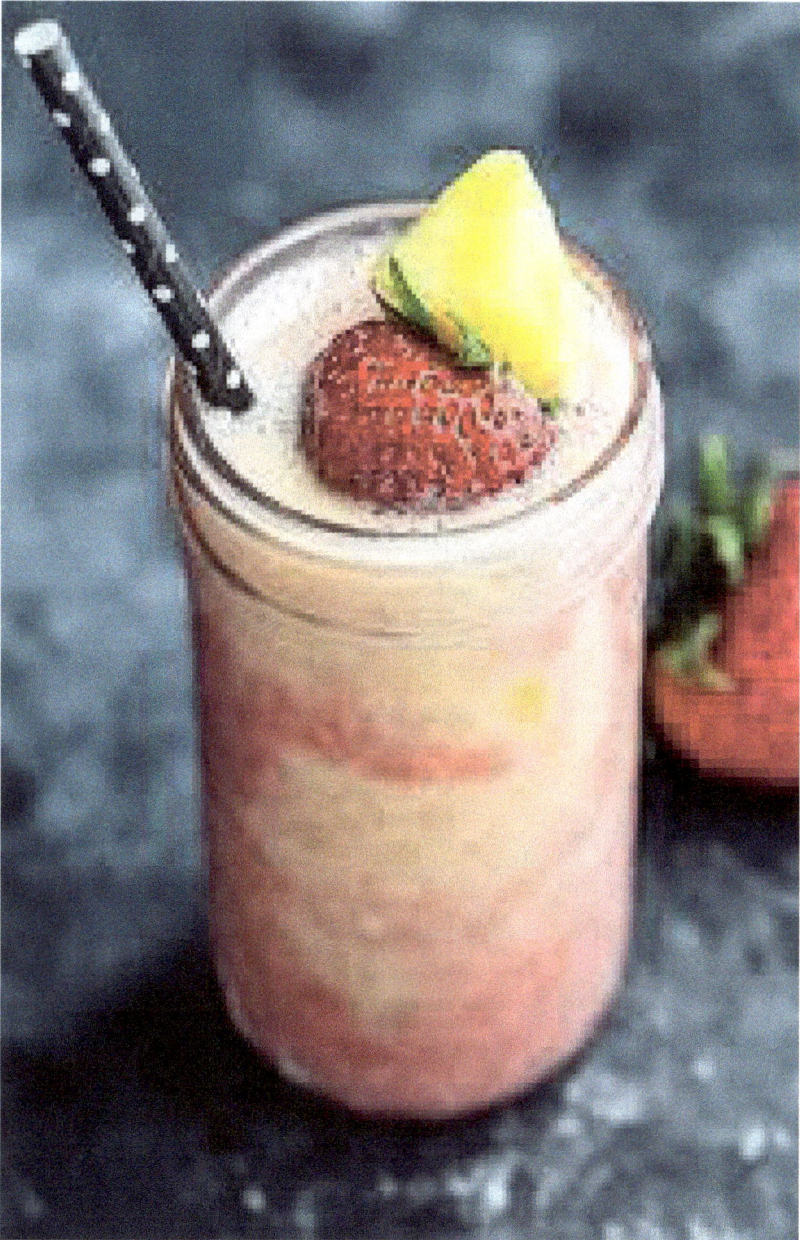

Preparation Time: 7 minutes

Cooking Time: 0 minute

Servings: 2

Ingredients :

- 1 cup strawberries
- 1 cup pineapple, chopped
- ¾ cup almond milk
- 1 tablespoon almond butter

Directions:

1. Add all Ingredients to a blender.

2. Blend until smooth.

3. Add more almond milk until it reaches your desired consistency.

4. Chill before serving.

Nutrition:

255 Calories

39g Carbohydrate

5.6g Protein

Cantaloupe Smoothie

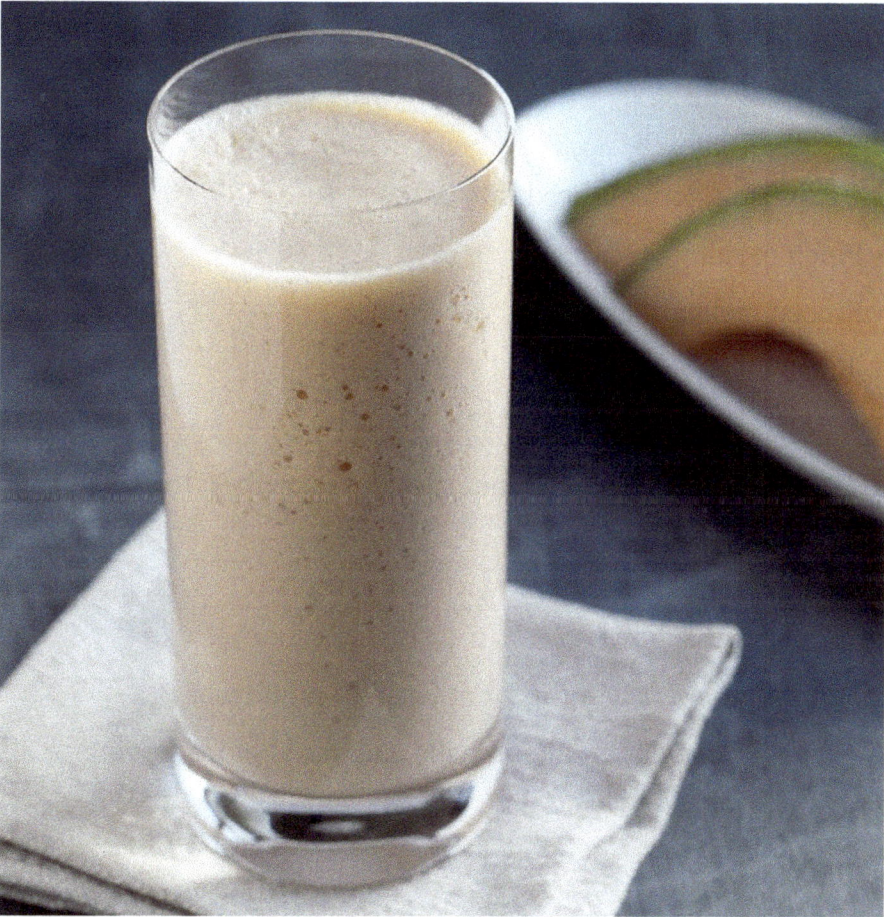

Preparation Time: 11 minutes

Cooking Time: 0 minute

Servings: 2

Ingredients :

- ¾ cup carrot juice
- 4 cups cantaloupe, sliced into cubes
- Pinch of salt
- Frozen melon balls
- Fresh basil

Directions:

1. Add the carrot juice and cantaloupe cubes to a blender. Sprinkle with salt.

2. Process until smooth.

3. Transfer to a bowl.

4. Chill in the refrigerator for at least 30 minutes.

5. Top with the frozen melon balls and basil before serving.

Nutrition:

135 Calories

31g Carbohydrate

3.4g Protein

Berry Smoothie with Mint

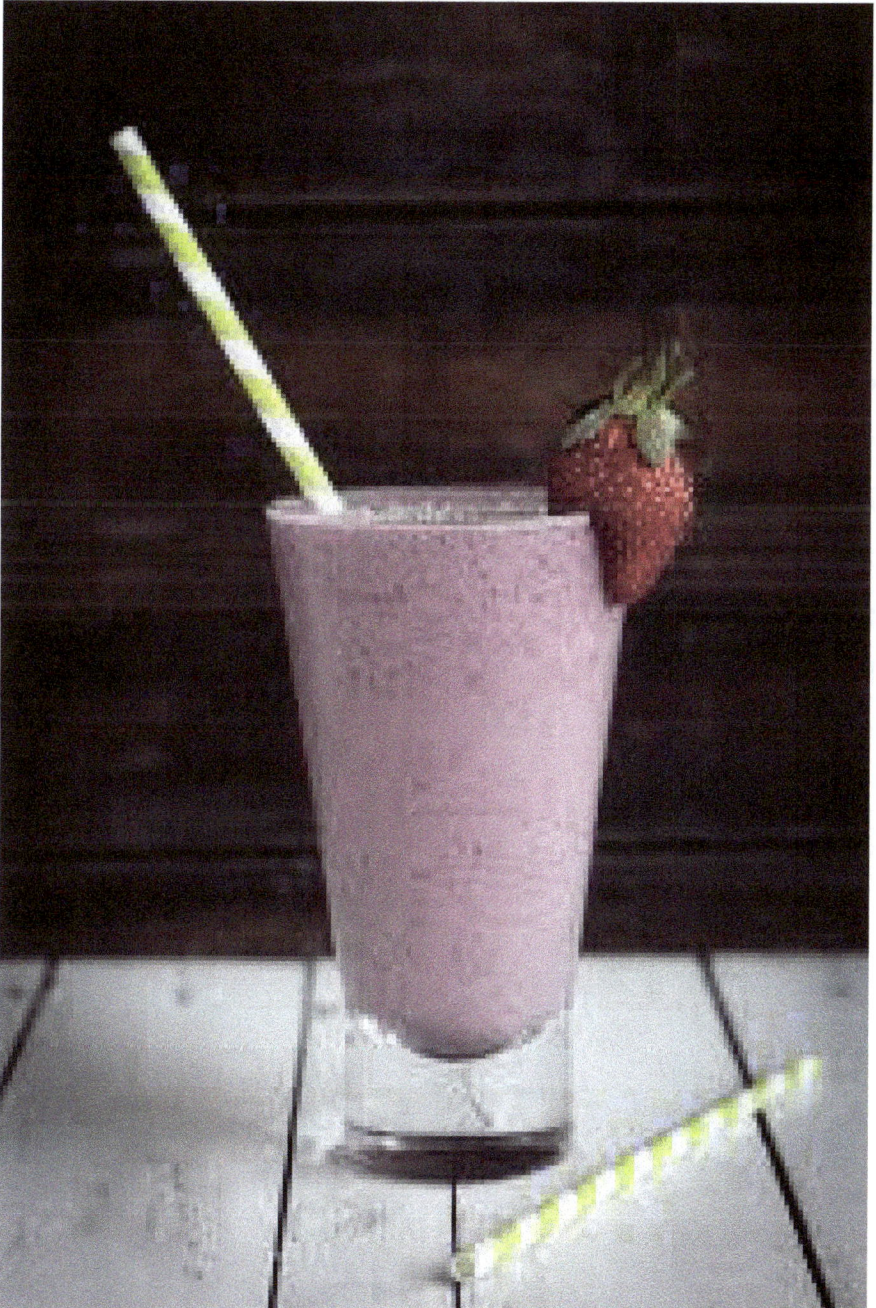

Preparation Time: 7 minutes

Cooking Time: 0 minute

Servings: 2

Ingredients :

- ¼ cup orange juice
- ½ cup blueberries
- ½ cup blackberries
- 1 cup reduced-fat plain kefir
- 1 tablespoon honey
- 2 tablespoons fresh mint leaves

Directions:

1. Add all the Ingredients to a blender.

2. Blend until smooth.

Nutrition:

137 Calories

27g Carbohydrate

6g Protein

Green Smoothie

Preparation Time: 12 minutes

Cooking Time: 0 minute

Servings: 2

Ingredients :

- 1 cup vanilla almond milk (unsweetened)
- ¼ ripe avocado, chopped
- 1 cup kale, chopped
- 1 banana
- 2 teaspoons honey
- 1 tablespoon chia seeds
- 1 cup ice cubes

Directions:

1. Combine all the Ingredients in a blender.

2. Process until creamy.

Nutrition:

343 Calories

14.7g Carbohydrate

5.9g Protein

Banana, Cauliflower & Berry Smoothie

Preparation Time: 9 minutes

Cooking Time: 0 minute

Servings: 2

Ingredients :

- 2 cups almond milk (unsweetened)
- 1 cup banana, sliced
- ½ cup blueberries
- ½ cup blackberries
- 1 cup cauliflower rice
- 2 teaspoons maple syrup

Directions:

1. Pour almond milk into a blender.

2. Stir in the rest of the Ingredients.

3. Process until smooth.

4. Chill before serving.

Nutrition:

149 Calories

29g Carbohydrate

3g Protein

Berry & Spinach Smoothie

Preparation Time: 11 minutes

Cooking Time: 0 minute

Servings: 2

Ingredients :

- 2 cups strawberries

- 1 cup raspberries

- 1 cup blueberries

- 1 cup fresh baby spinach leaves

- 1 cup pomegranate juice

- 3 tablespoons milk powder (unsweetened)

Directions:

1. Mix all the Ingredients in a blender.

2. Blend until smooth.

3. Chill before serving.

Nutrition:

118 Calories

25.7g Carbohydrate

4.6g Protein

Peanut Butter Smoothie with Blueberries

Preparation Time: 12 minutes

Cooking Time: 0 minute

Servings: 2

Ingredients :

• 2 tablespoons creamy peanut butter

• 1 cup vanilla almond milk (unsweetened)

• 6 oz. soft silken tofu

• ½ cup grape juice

• 1 cup blueberries

• Crushed ice

Directions:

1. Mix all the Ingredients in a blender.

2. Process until smooth.

Nutrition:

247 Calories

30g Carbohydrate

10.7g Protein

Peach & Apricot Smoothie

Preparation Time: 11 minutes

Cooking Time: 0 minute

Servings: 2

Ingredients :

- 1 cup almond milk (unsweetened)
- 1 teaspoon honey
- ½ cup apricots, sliced
- ½ cup peaches, sliced
- ½ cup carrot, chopped
- 1 teaspoon vanilla extract

Directions:

1. Mix milk and honey.

2. Pour into a blender.

3. Add the apricots, peaches and carrots.

4. Stir in the vanilla.

5. Blend until smooth.

Nutrition:

153 Calories

30g Carbohydrate

32.6g Protein

Tropical Smoothie

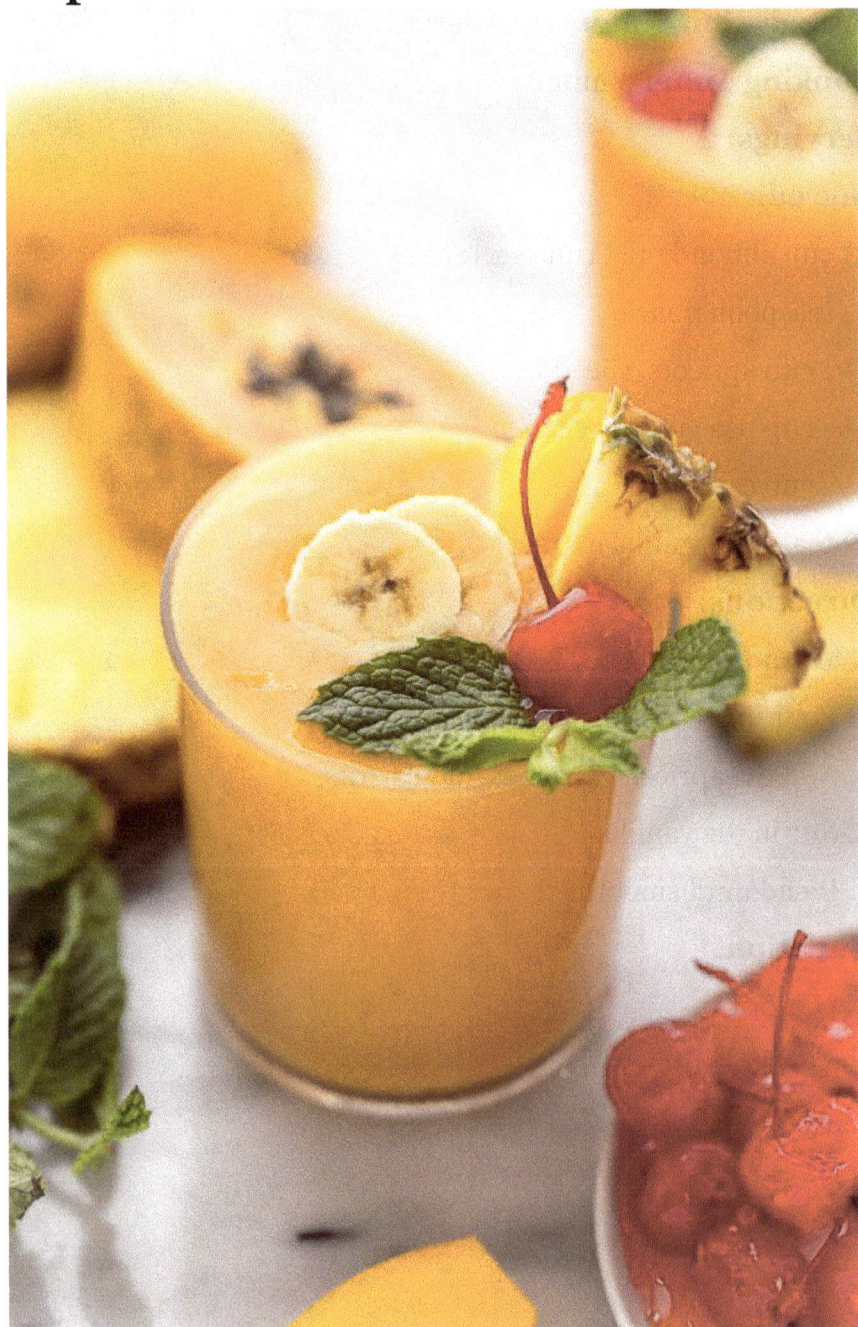

Preparation Time: 8 minutes

Cooking Time: 0 minute

Servings: 2

Ingredients :

- 1 banana, sliced
- 1 cup mango, sliced
- 1 cup pineapple, sliced
- 1 cup peaches, sliced
- 6 oz. nonfat coconut yogurt
- Pineapple wedges

Directions:

1. Freeze the fruit slices for 30 minutes.

2. Transfer to a blender.

3. Stir in the rest of the Ingredients except pineapple wedges.

4. Process until smooth.

5. Garnish with pineapple wedges.

Nutrition:

102 Calories

22.6g Carbohydrate

2.5g Protein

Banana & Strawberry Smoothie

Preparation Time: 7 minutes

Cooking Time: 0 minute

Servings: 2

Ingredients :

- 1 banana, sliced
- 4 cups fresh strawberries, sliced
- 1 cup ice cubes
- 6 oz. yogurt
- 1 kiwi fruit, sliced

Directions:

1. Add banana, strawberries, ice cubes and yogurt in a blender.

2. Blend until smooth.

3. Garnish with kiwi fruit slices and serve.

Nutrition:

54 Calories

11.8g Carbohydrate

1.7g Protein

Cantaloupe & Papaya Smoothie

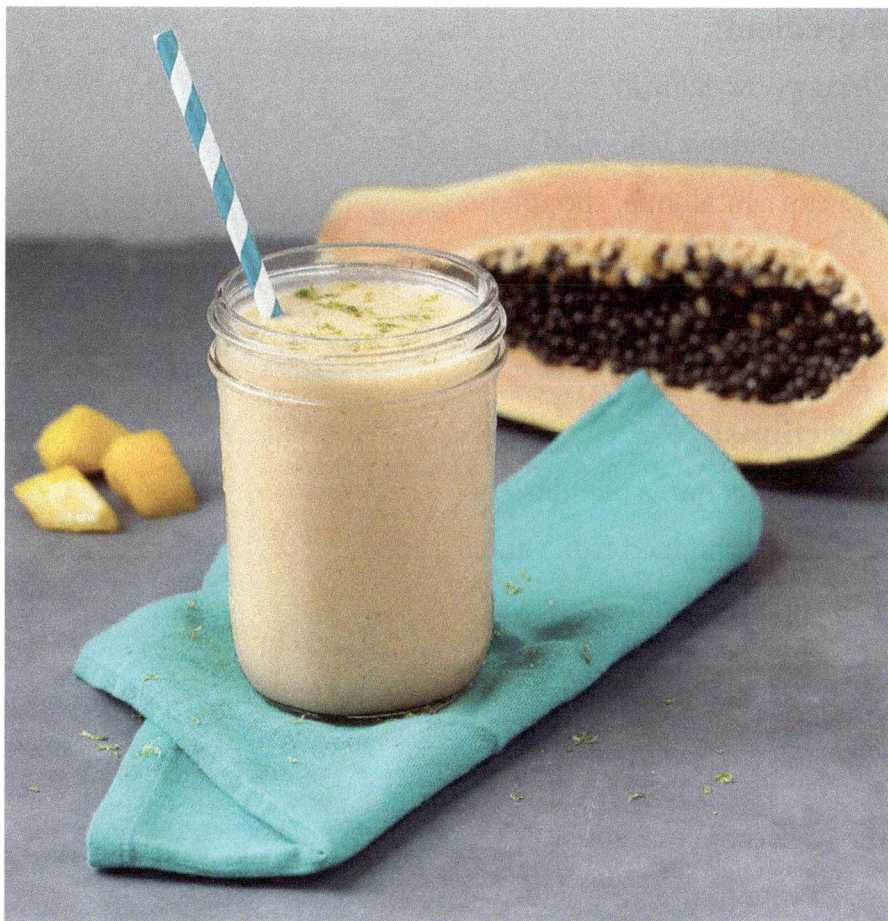

Preparation Time: 9 minutes

Cooking Time: 0 minute

Servings: 2

Ingredients :

- ¾ cup low-fat milk
- ½ cup papaya, chopped
- ½ cup cantaloupe, chopped
- ½ cup mango, cubed
- 4 ice cubes
- Lime zest

Directions:

1. Pour milk into a blender.

2. Add the chopped fruits and ice cubes.

3. Blend until smooth.

4. Garnish with lime zest and serve.

Nutrition:

207 Calories

18. 4g Carbohydrate

7. 7g Protein

www.ingramcontent.com/pod-product-compliance
Lightning Source LLC
Chambersburg PA
CBHW050755030426
42336CB00012B/1836